Suture and Surgical Hemostasis
A Pocket Guide

Suture and Surgical Hemostasis
A Pocket Guide

Rebecca Pieknik, CST/CSA, MS

SAUNDERS

ELSEVIER

SAUNDERS
ELSEVIER

11830 Westline Industrial Drive
St. Louis, Missouri 63146

SUTURE AND SURGICAL HEMOSTASIS: A POCKET GUIDE
ISBN-13: 978-1-4160-2247-3
ISBN-10: 1-4160-2247-3

Notice

Knowledge and best practice in this field are constantly changing. As new research and experience broaden our knowledge, changes in practice, treatment and drug therapy may become necessary or appropriate. Readers are advised to check the most current information provided (i) on procedures featured or (ii) by the manufacturer of each product to be administered, to verify the recommended dose or formula, the method and duration of administration, and contraindications. It is the responsibility of the practitioner, relying on their own experience and knowledge of the patient, to make diagnoses, to determine dosages and the best treatment for each individual patient, and to take all appropriate safety precautions. To the fullest extent of the law, neither the Publisher nor the Author assumes any liability for any injury and/or damage to persons or property arising out or related to any use of the material contained in this book.

ISBN-13: 978-1-4160-2247-3
ISBN-10: 1-4160-2247-3

Acquisitions Editor: Michael Ledbetter
Developmental Editor: Celeste Clingan
Publishing Services Manager: Pat Joiner
Project Manager: Jennifer Clark
Designer: Andrea Lutes

Printed in India
Last digit is the print number: 13

Working together to grow
libraries in developing countries

www.elsevier.com | www.bookaid.org | www.sabre.org

ELSEVIER   BOOK AID International   Sabre Foundation

I dedicate this book to Chris Keegan and Kathy Snyder for their continuous encouragement and support, and to my children April and Kevin, whose patience and understanding made this book possible.

Introduction

This suture book was written for those who want to better understand suture usage in closing wounds, tissue repair, and wound healing. One goal of suturing is to restore the continuity, integrity, and appearance to the tissue, and a person working in this discipline should have a basic understanding of suture and its application. Also, surgical technology students can use this book to enhance their knowledge and understanding of the characteristics of suture material used by surgeons to assist wound and tissue closure.

Contents

Wounds

CHAPTER 1

Anatomy of the Skin

To fully understand the pathophysiologic outcomes of disruptions in the integrity of skin, it is important to appreciate the anatomy of uninterrupted skin and tissue. The skin is part of the **integumentary** system and is also identified as the **cutaneous** membrane. Skin is vital to our existence and has several functions including the following:

1. **Protection.** The skin provides a physical obstacle from the external environment such as abrasions, dehydration, bacterial invasion, and ultraviolet rays.
2. **Excretion.** Perspiration by sweat glands eliminates waste material, salt, and water.
3. **Temperature Regulation.** During periods of excessive exercise, heat produced by the body is secreted through perspiration that helps lower the body temperature. During extreme heat loss, blood vessels near the surface constrict to reduce that heat loss.
4. **Sensory Perception.** The skin contains nerve endings that are receptors for pain, touch, and pressure.

5. **Synthesis of Vitamin D.** Exposure to ultraviolet radiation transforms molecules in the skin into vitamin D.

The Formation of Skin Layers

The skin varies in thickness according to location. It is thickest on the soles of our feet, where it may be as much as 6 mm in thickness, and thinnest on the eyelids, ear drums, and external genitalia, where it measures as little as 0.5 mm in depth. It consists of two main layers, the epidermis and the dermis (Fig. 1-1).

Epidermis

The epidermis is produced from stratified squamous epithelium cells, leaving it deficient of nerves, as well as blood vessels. In certain locations the epidermis consists of four or five layers (Fig. 1-2).

Dermis

Collagen and elastic fibers in the dermis layer are fibrous protein deposited by fibroblasts, and the **intrinsic** strength of these structures is what holds people together. The dermis attaches the epidermis to underlying tissue within its irregular surface by the papillae of the dermis passing in

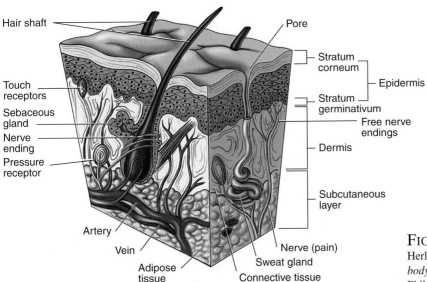

FIGURE **1-1** The skin. (From Herlihy B, Maebius NK: *The human body in health and illness*, ed 2, Philadelphia, 2003, Saunders.)

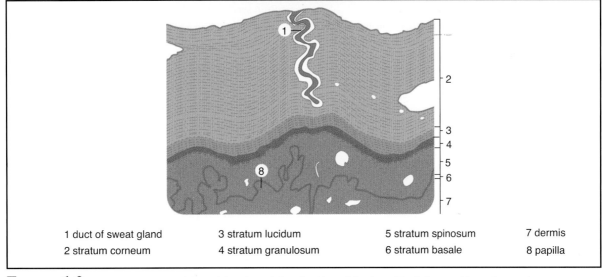

FIGURE **1-2** Photomicrograph of the epidermis and dermis. (From Morrison M: *Colour guide to the nursing management of chronic wounds*, ed 2, St Louis, 1996, Mosby.)

1 duct of sweat gland 3 stratum lucidum 5 stratum spinosum 7 dermis
2 stratum corneum 4 stratum granulosum 6 stratum basale 8 papilla

between the irregular spaces of the epidermis binding the two layers together. The dermis is loose, connective tissue and contains nerves, blood vessels, and **sebaceous** and **sudoriferous** glands. Epidermal ridges produce finger and toe prints that are unique to each person. The dermis is considered the main layer in wound repair and tissue healing (Fig. 1-3).

Subcutaneous Layer

The subcutaneous layer or superficial fascia consists primarily of loose connective and **adipose** tissue. Adipose tissue acts as a heat insulator and a storage site for fat (Fig. 1-4). The amount of adipose tissue varies among individuals and in different regions of the body. For example, adipose is thick over the abdomen but totally absent in the eyelids. The subcutaneous layer also contains the major blood vessels that supply the skin.

Fascia

The fascia is fibrous tissue that sustains the superficial skin layers and encloses the muscle (Fig. 1-5). Fascia is directly below the subcutaneous layer and is the point at which local anesthetic should be injected. Sensory nerve fibers are located here and the anesthetic is easily absorbed. Adipose occupies areolar spaces of the fascia accounting for the pliability that allows vessels, nerves, and lymphatic to pass through.

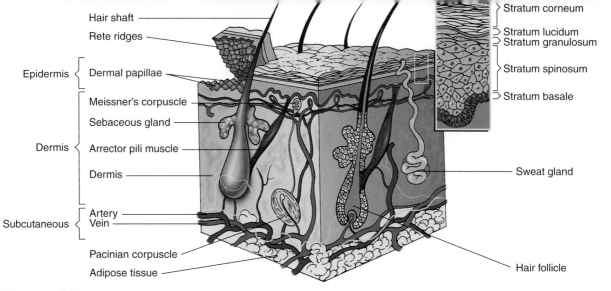

FIGURE **1-3** Anatomy of the skin. (From Linton AD, Maebius NK: *Introduction to medical-surgical nursing,* ed 3, Philadelphia, 2003, Saunders.)

Wounds

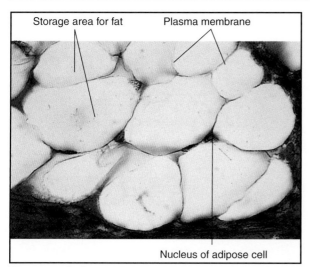

FIGURE **1-4** Adipose tissue. (From Thibodeau GA, Patton KT: *Structure and function of the body,* ed 12, St Louis, 2004, Mosby.)

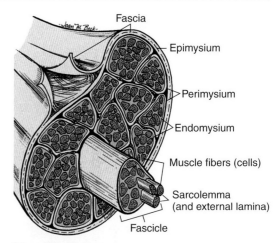

FIGURE **1-5** Anterior and posterior fascia. (From Lindsay DT: *Functional Human Anatomy*, St. Louis, 1996, Mosby.)

Accessory Structures

The accessory structures are developed from the epidermis. These structures originate in either the dermis or subcutaneous layer because they stem from the inward growth of the epidermis.

Hair is produced from **keratinized** cells and contains a shaft and a root. The shaft is the portion above the skin surface. The root is located below the skin surface in a hair follicle. Each hair follicle contains an **arrector pili** muscle that is attached to the follicle and the papillary layer of the dermis. When a person is frightened or cold, the arrector pili muscle will contract causing goose bumps and the hair to stand on end. Hair can be found on most body surfaces except the palms of the hands, soles of the feet, nipples, lips, and portions of the external genitalia.

Nails are composed of hard keratinized cells and cover the dorsal surface of the distal phalanges. A nail consists of a body and a root. Nails are colorless but appear pink due to blood vessels near the surface. The whitish crescent shape area of the nail is called the **lunula** (Fig. 1-6). The nails will appear bluish in persons that are suffering from **cyanosis** or severe anemia. Sebaceous glands are the oil-producing glands that empty into hair follicles. The oily secretion is called **sebum** and this helps keep the hair and skin pliable and soft. The palms and soles lack sebaceous glands but they are abundant on the scalp and face and natural body orifices. **Ceruminous** glands are modified sweat glands that produce a waxy substance known as cerumen. This protects the auditory canal from foreign substances. Cerumen is also known as earwax.

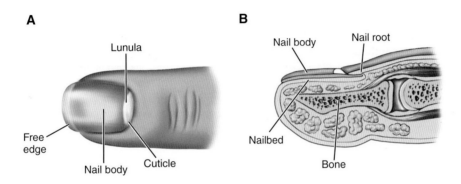

FIGURE **1-6** Structure of nails. (From Herlihy B, Maebius N: *The human body in health and illness*, ed 1, Philadelphia, 2000, Saunders.)

Wounds

Wounds are of three types, and they each occur differently. A wound may occur accidentally (traumatic), deliberately (surgical), or as a chronic-condition (pathophysiologic) disease process such as in a diabetic ulcer (Fig. 1-7, *A* through *C*).

Regardless of how it occurred, a wound is a disruption of tissue integrity. Various methods may be necessary to approximate a wound for proper healing including sutures, clips, staples, skin closure strips, or topical adhesives (Fig. 1-8, *A* through *D*).

Classification of Wounds

Wounds are classified on the basis of a clinical estimation of microbial contamination and the possible risk of infection. The Centers for Disease Control and Prevention (CDC) recommends four surgical wound classifications: clean, clean contaminated, contaminated, and dirty (Box 1-1). Operative wounds fall into these four distinct categories:

Class I: Clean (75% of surgical wounds fall into this category)

- No break in aseptic technique
- Incision is made under sterile conditions and is not predisposed to infection
- Primary closure

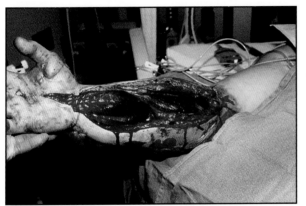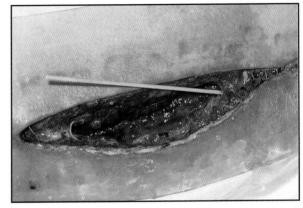

A   B

FIGURE 1-7 Types of wounds. **A,** Traumatic; **B,** Surgical; **C,** Pathophysiological (pressure ulcer). (*B* and *C* from Perry AG, Potter PA: *Clinical nursing skills & technology,* ed 6, St Louis, 2006, Mosby.)   *Continued*

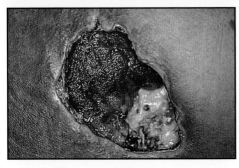

FIGURE **1-7** *Continued*

Box 1-1
Classification of Wounds

A: Class I—Clean
B: Class II—Clean contaminated
C: Class III—Contaminated
D: Class IV—Dirty/Infected

- No wound drain
- No entry into the oropharyngeal cavity, respiratory, alimentary, or genitourinary tracts

Class II: Clean Contaminated
- Minor break in aseptic technique transpired
- Respiratory, alimentary, or genitourinary tracts are entered under controlled circumstances
- Primary closure
- Wound is drained

Class III: Contaminated
- Fresh traumatic wounds
- Major breaks in sterile technique
- Acute inflammation present
- Gross spillage from gastrointestinal tract
- Infection from the genitourinary or biliary tract

Class IV: Dirty/Infected
- Old traumatic wounds or abscesses
- Perforated viscera
- Infection present at time of surgery

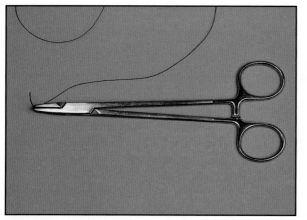 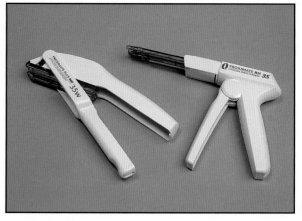

FIGURE **1-8** Types of wound closures. **A,** Suture. **B,** Staples. (Courtesy of Ethicon, Inc., Somerville, NJ.) *Continued*

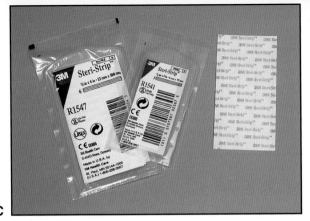

C

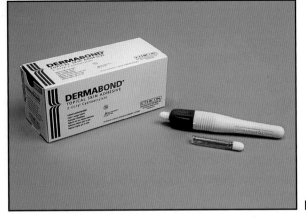

D

FIGURE **1-8** *Continued* **C,** Skin closure strips. **D,** Topical adhesives. (Courtesy of Ethicon, Inc., Somerville, NJ.)

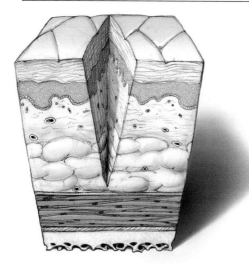

FIGURE **1-9** Surgical incision. (From Sherris D, Kern E: *Essential surgical skills*, ed 2, Philadelphia, 2004, Saunders.)

Intentional Wounds

The surgical site is an intentional wound. It can be an incision or an excision (Fig. 1-9). A primary incision is a cut into the skin made with a sterile scalpel. Excision is the removal of tissue by means of a scalpel, scissors, or thermal instrument such as an electrocautery device.

Occlusion banding is another means of an intentional wound. Hemorrhoid ligation results in ischemia of the hemorrhoid by means of banding. Fallopian tubes are also banded to interrupt the continuity of the lumen of the tube.

Chemicals, an uncommon form of an intentional wound, are applied to skin or other tissue surfaces to denude the area. The chemical process causes inflammation and reepithelialization to the skin surface as in a facial peel.

Unintentional Wounds

Following traumatic injury, preservation of life is the first critical concern. Traumatic wounds are also classified in several different categories.

Closed Wound

The skin remains intact, and underlying tissues are injured. A **hematoma** of blood and serum under the epidermis of the skin and simple fractures are considered closed wounds.

Open Wound

The skin is broken by abrasion, laceration, or penetration.

Simple Wound

The integrity of the skin is traumatized without loss or destruction of tissue and without the presence of a foreign body in the wound.

Complicated Wound

Tissue is lost or destroyed by means of a crush, burn, or foreign body in the wound. A foreign body is not removed until exploration is done and the wound is stabilized to prevent further injury. The wound may be closed by second or third intention depending on the amount of trauma to the tissue. Foreign objects such as bullets are secured for evidence (Fig. 1-10).

Clean Wound

The wound will heal by first intention with approximation of tissue and wound edges. Care is taken to assure a cosmetic closure, as well as preservation of normal function to the tissue.

Contaminated Wound

A contaminated wound occurs when a dirty object penetrates the integrity of the skin and tissues. Microorganisms multiply quickly, resulting in necessary debridement of tissue to remove devitalized tissue. Infection can set in within 6 hours of the initial injury. **Tetanus** can occur in deep wounds contaminated by soil or feces; therefore the patient's history should be assessed for tetanus immunization.

Delayed Full-Thickness Injury

A delayed, full-thickness injury is caused by industrial accidents including crush injuries and deep injection of substances. The full extent of damage may not be apparent for several days after the initial injury. Deep tissue **necrosis** can occur from electrocution or lightning several days after the initial injury (Fig. 1-11).

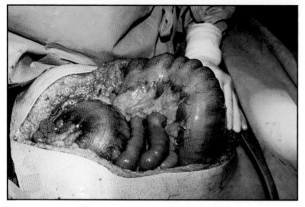

FIGURE **1-10** Complicated wound.

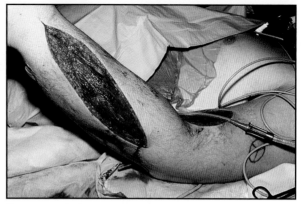

FIGURE **1-11** Full-thickness injury.

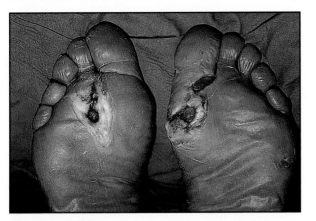

FIGURE **1-12** Chronic wound. (From Callen J, Greer K, Paller A, Swinyer L: *Color atlas of dermatology,* ed 2, Philadelphia, 1999, Saunders.)

Chronic Wounds

Chronic wounds are caused by pressure sores and **decubitus** ulcers due to compromised circulation over bony prominences or pressure points. Chronic wounds could result from an underlying condition. Venous stasis or arterial deficiency in the lower extremities may cause the development of chronic skin ulcers. Chronic wounds have tissue loss and may have heavy bacterial contamination. Failure of a wound to heal by second intention and granulated tissue formation might require debridement followed by skin grafting (Fig. 1-12).

CHAPTER 2

Wound Healing

Wound Healing

Tissue loss, contamination or infection, and damage to the tissue are determining factors of wound closure. The process of wound healing is related to whether the wound is closed or left open to heal.

Primary Intention (First Intention)

Healing through primary intention occurs when a wound is created aseptically with minimal tissue damage (Fig. 2-1). Healing through primary intention takes place by the following:
- No tissue loss
- Tissue edges are approximated with suture, staples, wound sealant, or steri strips
- Minimal or no postoperative swelling
- No contamination or infection

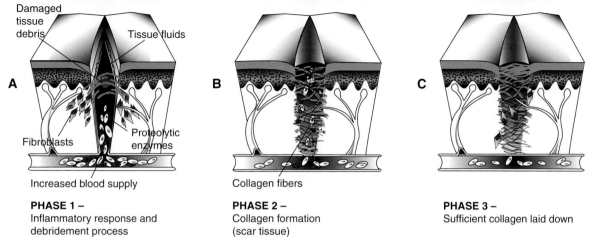

PHASE 1 –
Inflammatory response and
debridement process

PHASE 2 –
Collagen formation
(scar tissue)

PHASE 3 –
Sufficient collagen laid down

FIGURE 2-1 **A,** Phase 1. **B,** Phase 2. **C,** Phase 3. (From Ethicon: *Wound closure manual,* Somerville, NJ, 2004, Ethicon.)

- No dead space or separation of wound edges
- Minimal scar formation

There are several phases of would healing by primary (first) intention.

Phase I: The Inflammatory or Lag Phase (Days 1 to 5)

This stage begins immediately after the injury. Fluids that contain blood, lymph, and fibrin begin clotting and bind the cut edges together. A scab forms over the surface to seal in those fluids and prevent microbials from entering the wound. Inflammation presents as localized edema, pain, fever, and redness around the injury. **Leukocytes** accumulate to fight bacteria in the wound, and **phagocytosis** aids in removing damaged tissue. Basal cells from the skin edges migrate over the incision, closing the surface of the wound. **Fibroblasts** located in deep tissue begin the reconstruction of nonepithelial tissue.

Phase II: Proliferation Phase (Days 5 to 14)

This stage begins around the third day of the injury, overlapping the first phase of healing. Fibroblasts multiply quickly, drawing the wound edges together. Enzymes are released from blood and cells in surrounding tissue, and fibroblasts secrete collagen (fibrin, fibronectin) that forms into fibers to give the wound 25% to 30% of its tensile strength.

Phase III: Maturation/Remodeling (Day 14 through Complete Healing)

From day 14 until healing is complete, the wound undergoes a slow, constant change as scar tissue changes, increasing tensile strength. As collagen density increases, vascularity decreases and the scar fades. Skin only regains 70% to 90% of its original strength.

Secondary Intention (Granulation)

If the wound fails to heal by primary union, it is left open and allowed to heal from the inside toward the outer surface. Healing by second intention may be caused by infection, excessive trauma, tissue loss, or inability to reapproximate the tissue (Fig. 2-2). Considerations of second intention include the following:

- The wound may be left open to heal from the inner layer to outer surface
- Granulation tissue forms, aiding in wound closure by contraction
- It is a slower process than first intention

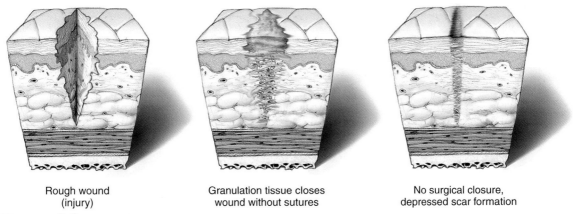

Rough wound
(injury)

Granulation tissue closes
wound without sutures

No surgical closure,
depressed scar formation

FIGURE 2-2 Healing by second intention. (From Sherris DA, Kern EB: *Essential surgical skills,* ed 2, Philadelphia, 2004, Saunders.)

Third Intention (Tertiary)

Third intention is also referred to as *delayed primary closure.* Healing occurs when two surfaces of granulation tissue are joined. This is the favored method for contaminated, dirty, or infected traumatic wounds with tissue loss. The surgical wound is debrided and purposely left open to heal by third intention (Fig. 2-3). Considerations include the following:

- Intentionally delayed by 3 or more days
- May require a primary and secondary suture line
- Removal of an inflamed organ
- Heavy contamination of the wound

Factors of Wound Healing

Factors that affect wound healing are influenced by the patient's overall health status. These factors should be taken into consideration by the surgical team.

- Age: With aging, skin and muscle tissue may lose their tone and elasticity. Metabolism slows, and circulation may be compromised.
- Weight: Excess fat surrounding the wound may prevent a good wound closure. To minimize **dead space**, the surgeon may place drains and suture in subcutaneous fat. Of all the tissues, adipose tissue is the most vulnerable to trauma and infection due to poor vascularity.

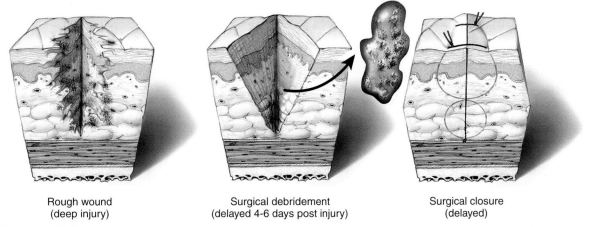

Rough wound
(deep injury)

Surgical debridement
(delayed 4-6 days post injury)

Surgical closure
(delayed)

FIGURE **2-3** Healing by third intention. (From Sherris DA, Kern EB: *Essential surgical skills,* ed 2, Philadelphia, 2004, Saunders.)

- Nutritional status: Wound healing can be impaired by deficiencies in carbohydrates; proteins; zinc; and vitamins A, B, and C. Adequate nutrition is imperative to support cellular growth.
- Dehydration: Electrolyte imbalance may affect cardiac function, kidney function, cellular metabolism, oxygenation of the blood, and hormonal function, and any discrepancies in these processes may impair the healing process.
- Disease (chronic or acute): Any patient whose system is traumatized by chronic illness such as endocrine disorders, diabetes, malignancies, localized infection, or debilitating disease will experience a negative impact on the healing response.
- Inadequate blood supply: Oxygen is essential for cell survival and healing. Skin healing occurs fastest in the face and neck, where there is great vascularity, and slowest in the extremities. Any condition that compromises blood flow to the wound will impede the healing process.
- Radiation exposure: Large doses of radiation treatment may decrease blood supply to the irradiated tissue and impair healing.
- Immune responses: The immune response protects the patient from infection; any immunodeficiency may seriously influence the outcome of a surgical procedure. An allergy to suturing materials, latex, or metal alloys may also cause an immune response from the patient. This could obstruct the normal healing process.

Surgical Principles of Wound Healing

The surgeon's goal is to achieve wound closure with minimal defect and dysfunction. This can be achieved by understanding the biology of wound repair, which includes the response of living tissue to the injury. Other factors that influence wound healing are aspects of the surgical procedure that can be controlled by the surgical team. These include the following:

- Length and direction of the incision—wounds naturally heal from side-to-side, not end-to-end.
- Dissection technique—An incision with an evenly applied clean stroke of pressure will assist wound closure.
- Tissue handling—keeping tissue trauma to a minimum with careful handling will prevent complications.
- Maintaining moisture in the tissue—Covering exposed areas with saline-soaked sponges or periodically irrigating the wound will prevent tissues from drying out and enhances proper wound closure.
- Hemostasis—Achieving hemostasis through mechanical, thermal, and chemical methods will decrease the flow of blood into the wound site. Attaining complete hemostasis will eliminate the formation of postoperative hematomas.
- Removal of necrotic tissue—Debridement of all devitalized tissue and removal of all foreign substances is imperative to good healing. Any presence of foreign material will increase the probability of infection.

- Choice of suture material—The choice of suture is based on each individual and will maximize the process of healing. The proper material will approximate tissue with little trauma, as well as eliminate dead space.
- Cellular response to suture material—Suture is considered a foreign object, and the tissue will react. Edema of the skin or subcutaneous tissues will develop; therefore the surgeon should consider this when placing tension on the wound closure.
- Elimination of dead space—This is one of the most critical aspects of wound closure. Dead space occurs from separation of wound edges that have not been correctly approximated or from air that remains trapped between the layers of the tissue. Serum or blood may collect, leading to the growth of microorganisms that cause infection. Inserting a drain or applying a pressure dressing will help eliminate dead space postoperatively.
- Wound stress—Any postoperative activity will place stress on the healing incision. Coughing, vomiting, voiding, or defecating will cause tension on abdominal fascia. Extremities may also experience stress during healing. Surgeons must ensure the approximated wound is adequately immobilized to prevent suture disruption.

Complications of Wound Healing

Whenever the integrity of the skin is compromised, the wound is subject to infection and complications. Many factors can influence wound healing including the following:

- **Dehiscence**: Partial or total separation of a surgical incision or rupture of a wound closure (Fig. 2-4, *A*). Dehiscence can lead to retrograde infection, peritonitis, or evisceration if it involves an abdominal incision.
- **Evisceration**: Protrusion of viscera through the abdominal cavity from a wound or surgical incision (Fig. 2-4, *B*). It is considered an emergency situation that requires immediate attention.
- **Hemorrhage**: A large amount of blood loss either internally or externally. Surgery is often necessary to achieve hemostasis.
- **Infection**: The invasion of a pathogenic microorganism that dominates the host. It results in increased morbidity and mortality. Antibiotics and possible additional surgery may be required (Fig. 2-5). Sutured wounds must be covered by a dressing to protect against infection from skin bacterial contamination.
- **Adhesion**: Scar tissue that binds together two anatomic surfaces that are normally separate from each other (Fig. 2-6). Adhesions are most commonly found in the abdomen, where they form after abdominal surgery, inflammation, or injury.
- **Herniation**: Protrusion of a body organ or portion of an organ through an abnormal opening in a membrane, muscle, or other tissue.

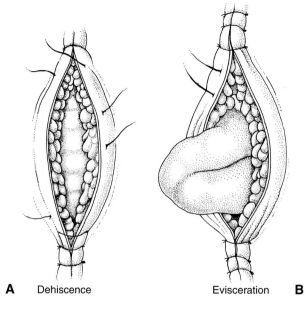

A Dehiscence   **B** Evisceration

FIGURE **2-4** Complications of wound healing. **A,** Dehiscence. **B,** Evisceration. (From Rothrock J: *Alexander's care of the patient in surgery,* ed 12, St Louis, 2002, Mosby.)

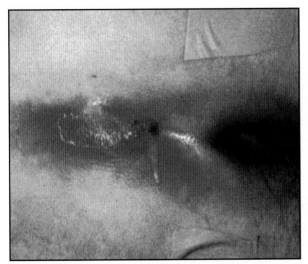

FIGURE **2-5** Infection. (From Morrison M: *Colour guide to the nursing management of chronic wounds,* ed 2, London, 1996, Mosby.)

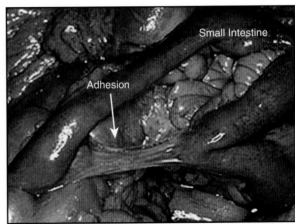

FIGURE **2-6** Adhesion. (From www.gihealth.com.)

- **Fistula**: An abnormal tract between two epithelium-lined surfaces that is open at both ends. It happens frequently after bladder, bowel, or pelvic surgeries (Fig. 2-7).
- **Sinus tract**: A tract between two epithelium lined surfaces that is open only at one end.
- **Suture complications**: Complications from suture often occur if there is failure for the tissue to absorb the suture material or if the suture causes a reaction or inflammation.
- **Keloid scar**: Formation of a hypertrophic scar that occurs most often in dark-skinned individuals (Fig. 2-8).

Tissue Layer Closure
Abdominal Closure

Abdominal wounds should be closed layer by layer. The type of closure may be more important than the type of suture used. The layers include peritoneum, fascia, muscle, subcutaneous, and skin.

Peritoneum

The peritoneum or thick membrane lining the abdominal cavity lies beneath the posterior fascia. The peritoneum is a thin layer. Some surgeons do not believe in closing this layer, while others believe that tissue should be put back the way it was found. If the posterior fascia is closed firmly,

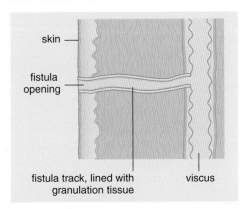

FIGURE 2-7 Fistula. (From Morrison M: *Colour guide to the nursing management of chronic wounds,* ed 2, London, 1996, Mosby.)

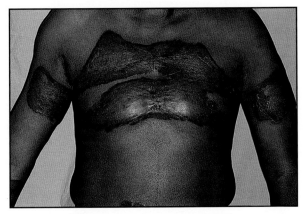

FIGURE 2-8 Keloid scar. (From Callen J: *Color atlas of dermatology,* ed 2, Philadelphia, 1999, Saunders.)

suturing the peritoneum will not prevent an incisional hernia. When a surgeon closes peritoneum, a continuous suture line with absorbable suture is often used. Interrupted sutures may also be used for this closure.

Fascia

Fascia is a strong layer of connective tissue that covers the muscle and is considered the main supportive structure of the body. The fatty superficial section is known as *Camper's fascia,* while the membranous deep part is called Scarpa's fascia. When closing the abdominal incision, the fascial sutures must hold the wound closed and help resist changes in intraabdominal pressure (Fig. 2-9). Occasionally a synthetic graft may be used for extra support if the fascia is absent or weak.

Muscle

Muscles are not typically closed because they do not tolerate suturing well. Muscles may be separated or cut and retracted. Avoiding interfering with the blood supply and nerve function of a muscle is always best. During closure, abdominal muscles are not sutured; the fascia (Scarpa's and transversalis fascia) surrounding the muscle is sutured instead (Fig. 2-10).

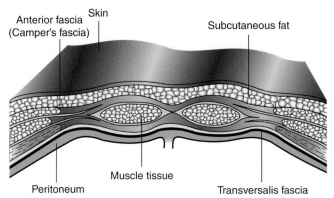

FIGURE **2-9** Fascia layer. (From Ethicon: *Wound closure manual,* Somerville, NJ, 2004, Ethicon.)

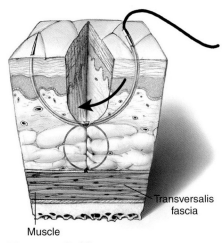

FIGURE **2-10** Closure of muscle layer. (From Sherris DA, Kern EB: *Essential surgical skills,* ed 2, Philadelphia, 2004, Saunders.)

A single-layer closure of both layers of abdominal wall fascia, abdominal muscles, peritoneum, and the anterior fascia layer is known as the *Smead Jones far and near technique.* This closure provides support for the healing process with a low incidence of wound disruption. The closure is done with a figure-of-eight stitch consisting of PDS II sutures or Vicryl. Monofilament Prolene suture will also provide strength, minimal tissue reactivity, and resistance to bacterial contamination, as does stainless steel, although Prolene is better tolerated.

Subcutaneous

Subcutaneous tissue does not handle suture well, either; however, many surgeons believe it is important to place sutures in subcutaneous tissue to eliminate dead space. Dead space is likely to occur in this type of tissue, so the wound must be thoroughly approximated (Fig. 2-11). Tissue fluids can accumulate in dead space, delaying the healing process. Absorbable suture such as Vicryl or plain gut is often chosen for the subcutaneous layer because it is absorbed by hydrolysis.

Skin Closure

Skin is composed of the epithelium and underlying dermis. It is tough, and a sharp cutting needle is essential for the stitch to minimize tissue trauma. If a nonabsorbable suture material is used, it is removed 3 to 10 days postoperatively. Because monofilament sutures provide less tissue reaction than multifilament sutures, they are the preferred choice of suture material. Nylon, polypropylene, or skin staples offer minimal tissue reaction. These may be placed with interrupted or continuous stitches (Fig. 2-12). The disadvantage to skin closure is that the wound scars more than with a subcuticular closure.

Subcuticular

The subcuticular layer of tough connective tissue will hold skin edges together, which induces minimal scarring. The surgeon uses continuous short lateral stitches just beneath the epithelial layer of skin in a line parallel to the skin. Absorbable sutures are most often used, although nonabsorbable sutures are an option. If nonabsorbable sutures are chosen, one end of the suture strand will protrude from each end of the incision and the surgeon may tie them together in a loop or tie each end outside the incision. To hold the closure in tight approximation and minimize scarring, skin closure tapes are used in conjunction with the subcuticular closure.

Some surgeons may choose to close both the subcuticular and epidermal layers to further minimize scarring.

Endoscopic Closure

Endoscopy may require the use of a suture ligature placed through a trocar cannula. Plastic delivery devices assist delivery of preknotted ligatures. Endoscopic sutures are available as ligatures and

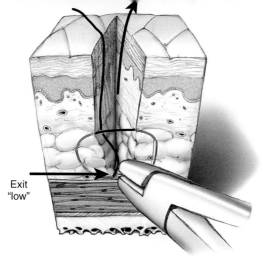

Exit "low"

Second bite – exit "low"

FIGURE **2-11** Subcutaneous closure. (From Sherris DA, Kern EB: *Essential surgical skills,* ed 2, Philadelphia, 2004, Saunders.)

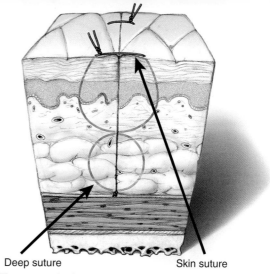

Deep suture

Skin suture

FIGURE **2-12** Skin closure with suture. (From Sherris DA, Kern EB: *Essential surgical skills,* ed 2, Philadelphia, 2004, Saunders.)

preknotted loops or with curved or straight, permanently swaged needles for use with the endoscope. Endoscopic ligatures are formed into loops before being passed through the endoscope. After the loop is placed around the vessel or tissue, the knot will be tightened. The ends of the suture are cut with endoscopic scissors and removed. Suture with permanently swaged-on needle are passed through a 3-mm suture introducer for a straight needle and an 8-mm suture introducer for a curved needle. Two methods are used to properly tie knots endoscopically.

1. **Extracorporeal** method. The swaged needle and suture ends are brought outside the body through a trocar. The needle is then cut and a loose knot is created. The knot is reintroduced into the body through the trocar with the use of a knot-sliding cannula. It is pushed into position and tightened against the tissue. The ends of the suture are cut close to the knot.

2. **Intracorporeal** method. The needle and suture are passed through the tissue with an endoscopic needle holder. Endoscopic instruments are used to tie the knot and cut the suture.

CHAPTER 3

Suture

History of Suture

References to suture date back to 2500 BC. Animal sinews such as tendons and ligaments and linen strips were the first recorded sutures used to bring wound edges together. Throughout the century, sheep gut intestines, and catgut along with cotton, leather, and horsehair were added to the selection of materials to close tissue. The science of suturing progressed slowly; patients succumbed to hemorrhage, pain, and infection due to the lack of sterile technique.

The nineteenth century saw sterile technique evolve as **Lister** first used carbolic acid solution and established the necessity of sterile surgical suture. Lister also used surgical gut as an absorbable suture material that was presented in sterile glass tubes. Suture material rapidly progressed with numerous materials such as gold, silver, metallic wire, gut, silk, cotton, linen, and tendons. The most commonly used sutures of the twentieth century included surgical gut, silk, and cotton. The latter part of the twentieth century saw the use of synthetic textiles such as nylon, polyester, polypropylene, and other polymer materials. In 1909 Davis and Geck perfected a method for sterilizing surgical gut and sealing it in glass tubes.

Definition of Suture

The word *suture* describes any material used to approximate tissue edges together or ligate blood vessels. A suture attached to a needle is referred to as a **stick tie** (Fig. 3-1). A **free tie** is a single strand of suture handed to the surgeon. When the free tie is placed on the tip of a forceps or instrument, it is considered a **tie on a passer** (Fig. 3-2). The choice of suture material should be based on the biologic reaction of the materials used, the tissue that is being sutured, and the characteristic of the wound. The tissue should be held in place until the **tensile strength** of the wound can withstand stress. Important considerations are the type of suture, knot, and type of stitch used to approximate the tissue.

The advancement of suture selection in the 1940s brought about uniform preparation and sterilization of suture materials, as well as specific sutures for specific specialties. In the 1950s, sutures with swaged-on or preattached needles were individually packaged in plastic wrappers and sterilized for passing onto the sterile field (Fig. 3-3). Synthetic, absorbable sutures were introduced in the 1960s. Synthetic sutures consisted of polyglycolic acid, which maintains high tensile strength and minimal tissue reaction. Today suture material is individually packaged and is sterilized by cobalt-60 irradiation or ethylene oxide gas. Steam sterilization is not a viable option. The protein in natural absorbable materials coagulates, and moisture and heat affect synthetic absorbable sutures. Only stainless steel suture material can be steam sterilized.

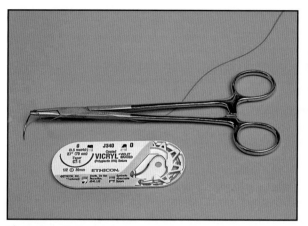

FIGURE **3-1** Stick tie. (Courtesy of Ethicon, Inc., Somerville, NJ.)

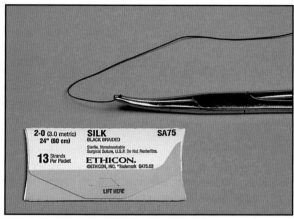

FIGURE **3-2** Tie on a passer. (Courtesy of Ethicon, Inc., Somerville, NJ.)

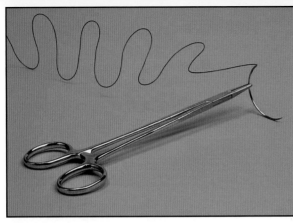

FIGURE **3-3** Swaged-on needle.

Characteristics of Suture Material

As technology advanced, suture material advanced as well. Unfortunately, the perfect suture still does not exist. If it did, it would be described as follows:

- Sterile and cost efficient
- Nonelectrolytic, noncapillary, nonallergenic, and noncarcinogenic
- Inert, as in stainless steel suture
- Easy to handle
- Capable of securely holding tissue layers throughout the wound-healing process
- Minimally reactive in tissue and not predisposed to bacterial growth
- Resistant to the shrinking tissue, as tissue heals
- Absorbed completely with minimal tissue reaction once the wound was healed

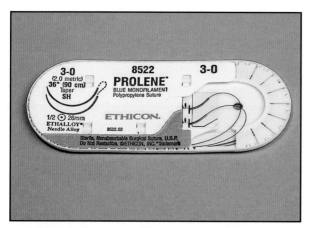

FIGURE **3-4** Inner package of suture material.
(Courtesy of Ethicon, Inc., Somerville, NJ.)

Presentation of Suture Material

Each suture package has two layers to allow for transfer
to the sterile field. The outer cover (dust cover) is made
of laminate backing that is heat sealed together. The
design of the inner package for absorbable sutures is
different from nonabsorbable sutures (Fig. 3-4). Because
absorbable sutures must be protected from moisture, the
sterile inner packets are **hermetically** sealed aluminum
foil cavities designed to tear with ease. The upper edge of
the sterile inner packet has a tear notch that provides
consistent opening. This allows easy access to the needle
set in the foam, which can be loaded for right-handed
surgeons. With Ethicon suture material, there is a slight
difference in the inner packet for the nonabsorbable
suture material. It has a midpeel opening in the packet
with an access flap that is lifted from the inner packet
and turned 180 degrees to expose the body of the needle
set in the foam. By rotating the access flap, the needle
can be armed from either side to accommodate right- or

left-handed surgeons. The needle is positioned in a manner that prevents kinking of the monofilament suture.

Presentation of Suture Material

For both absorbable and nonabsorbable sutures, systems have been designed to stabilize braided and monofilament sutures in their packets. For braided sutures, a rigid plastic container with a spiral **labyrinth** is specially designed for delivery of kink-free sutures. A suture is removed from the labyrinth in a manner that maintains its uniform configuration. The suture is swaged onto a needle set in the foam that protects the needle point and cutting edges. When a suture contains a swaged needle, the silhouette of the needle is pictured on the label along with the size and type of suture material. The memory of monofilament is so great that the shape of the suture conforms to the shape of the package.

Trauma to the suture by surgical instruments can seriously compromise suture **efficacy**. Grasping the suture with clamps and forceps, as well as running one's fingers along the strand, could damage or weaken the suture.

The coiled monofilament suture is wrapped around the four fixation pins in figure-of-eight–shaped loops that are secured in craft paper boards. Even after removing it from the package, the suture will take on a figure-of-eight shape. The monofilament suture must be straightened before

---

it is handed to the surgeon by applying force to both suture ends. This is known as "removing the memory from the suture."

Suture boxes may contain one, two, or three dozen packets of sterile suture material. The label on the box is usually color coded to the suture material (Fig. 3-5).

Surgeon Preference

Most surgeons have a personal preference for routinely using the same suture material. The surgeon attains skill, proficiency, and speed in handling by using the same suture material repetitively. The surgeon's knowledge of the physical characteristics of suture material plays a major role in suture choice. Requirements for wound support vary with each patient and are based on the type of procedure, the tissue involved, and the time needed for wound healing. A number of factors may influence the choice of materials:

- His or her area of specialization
- Wound closure experience during clinical training
- Professional experience in the operating room
- Knowledge of the healing characteristics of tissues and organs
- Knowledge of the physical and biologic characteristics of various suture material
- Patient factors (age, weight, overall health status, and presence of any infection)

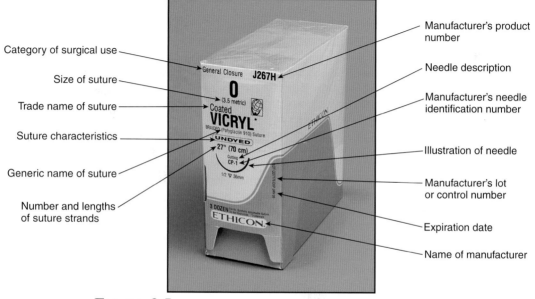

Category of surgical use — General Closure · **J267H** — Manufacturer's product number

Size of suture — **0** (3.5 metric) — Needle description

Trade name of suture — Coated **VICRYL** — Manufacturer's needle identification number

Suture characteristics — BRAIDED (Polyglactin 910) Suture · **UNDYED** — Illustration of needle

Generic name of suture — 27" (70 cm) · Cutting CP-1 · 1/2 ▽ 36mm — Manufacturer's lot or control number

Number and lengths of suture strands — 3 DOZEN — Expiration date

ETHICON — Name of manufacturer

FIGURE **3-5** Suture box. (Courtesy of Ethicon, Inc., Somerville, NJ.)

Suture Size

The U.S. Pharmacopeia (USP) defines the physical characteristics of suture material. The size of the suture refers to the diameter of the suture material. Suture sizes are selected on the basis of the tissue being sutured. Surgeons choose the smallest possible suture that will approximate the tissue while healing. This is why it is important to understand the tissue layers for wound closure. Choosing the smallest suture for the tissue approximation reduces the trauma as the suture passes through the tissue. Suture size is stated numerically and is based on a number chart. As the numbers increase, the diameter of the suture decreases. For example, size 4-0 is smaller than 3-0. The smaller the size, the less tensile strength the suture has.

The knot tensile strength is measured by the force in pounds a suture will withstand before it breaks when knotted. The tensile strength of the tissue to be sutured determines the size and tensile strength of the suture the surgeon uses. The tensile strength of the suture should never exceed the tensile strength of the tissue. The diameter size of stainless steel is determined by Brown and Sharpe (B & S) commercial wire gauge numbers. The largest suture is number 5, while the smallest suture size is 11-0. USP suture sizes #1 through 4-0 are most commonly used. The length of suture material ranges from 13 cm to 150 cm.

Suture Strands
Monofilament

Suture material is categorized by the number of strands it comprises. A single strand of material is considered a monofilament suture. A **monofilament** (Fig. 3-6) suture goes through tissue with less drag or resistance than multifilament. This is important when considering that organisms may cause suture line or wound infection. Because monofilament resists infection, it is often the choice in vascular surgery. The monofilament material also makes it easy to crush. Extreme care must be taken when using monofilament sutures. Suture boots (Fig. 3-7) placed on mosquito clamps protect the suture from being crushed if the surgeon wants the suture **tagged** or is using it to retract tissue. Examples of monofilament suture include Prolene and PDS II.

Multifilament

Multifilament sutures consist of several filaments or suture strands braided together. This allows for greater tensile strength, pliability, and flexibility of the suture. Multifilament sutures may be coated to help them pass through tissue with less drag (Fig. 3-8). Coated multifilament sutures work well for intestinal procedures. Because of the braiding, multifilament sutures allow for **wicking;** therefore it should never be used in the presence of infection. Wicking is a method by which an organism can enter the tissue. Examples of multifilament or braided suture include Vicryl and silk.

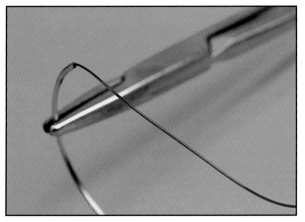

FIGURE **3-6** Monofilament suture.

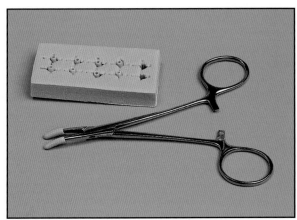

FIGURE **3-7** Suture boots.

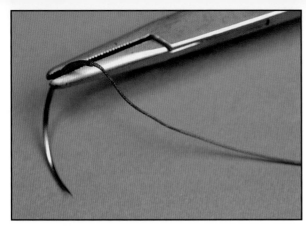

FIGURE **3-8** Multifilament suture.

Absorbable Suture Material

Suture material is categorized according to absorption rates. Absorbable sutures are designed to hold wound edges together until they have healed sufficiently to endure normal stress. Absorbable sutures are processed from the collagen of healthy mammals or from synthetic polymers. Natural absorbable sutures absorb quickly, while other sutures are coated purposely to lengthen their absorption time. Suture material may also be coated to improve handling properties or colored with FDA-approved dye to improve visibility for the surgeon. Plain gut and Vicryl would be examples of absorbable suture material.

Natural, absorbable sutures are digested by enzymes in the body that break sutures down, while synthetic absorbable sutures are broken down by **hydrolysis**—a process in which water slowly penetrates sutures and breaks down their polymer chain. During the first stage of

---

hydrolysis, tensile strength weakens in a slow, linear manner over several weeks. The second stage overlaps the first stage of hydrolysis and is distinguished by suture mass loss. Both stages show evidence of leukocytic cellular responses that remove cellular debris and suture material from the line of tissue approximation. Absorbable suture material may lose tensile strength rapidly while being absorbed slowly, or it can maintain tensile strength through wound healing and is then absorbed quickly. Absorbable suture material is completely dissolved without any of the suture remaining.

The absorption rate of suture material is affected by a patient's health status. If the patient has a fever, infection, or protein deficiency, the rate is accelerated. Postoperative complications can arise if sutures are wet or moist and may lead to the absorption process beginning prematurely.

Nonabsorbable Suture Material

Nonabsorbable suture material is not digested by the body's enzymes or hydrolyzed in body tissue. Instead, it is **encapsulated** in the tissue. Nonabsorbable suture material can be composed of single or multiple filaments of metal, synthetic, or organic fibers. Each strand is uniform in diameter throughout its length to correspond to USP standards. Stainless steel, nylon, and silk are nonabsorbable suture material.

Nonabsorbable sutures may be coated or uncoated, clear, or dyed to improve visibility. The following conditions obviously warrant nonabsorbable sutures:

- Skin closure—usually placed with interrupted stitches that are removed after healing has occurred
- Body cavities or vessels—these sutures remain permanently as the body encapsulates them (i.e., anastomosis of a vessel)
- Patient history—if there is a reaction to absorbable sutures, **keloidal** tendency, or tissue **hypertrophy**
- Prosthesis attachment—in cases of defibrillators, pacemakers, and MediPorts, these sutures remain indefinitely

Ligation of Vessels

Several methods can be used to **ligate** a vessel. Ligating involves occluding a vessel to prevent it from hemorrhaging when it is dissected. Vessels can either be occluded with stainless steel clips or ligated with suture material. Freehand ligatures are also referred to as "free ties" and are used for occluding vessels, ducts, or other structures. Nonneedled sutures or ties are available in standard lengths of 54 inches for absorbable and 60 inches for nonabsorbable sutures. Surgical technologists can cut suture strands into halves, thirds, or fourths. Suture ties (Fig. 3-9) are also available in precut lengths of 18-, 24-, and 30-inch strands.

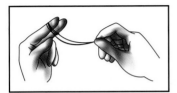

1. Prepare cut lengths of ligature material, coil around fingers of left hand, grasp free ends with right hand, and unwind to full length.

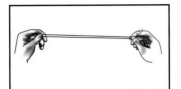

2. Maintain loop in left hand and two free ends in right hand. Gently pull the strand to straighten.

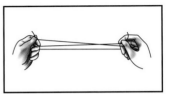

3. To make 1/3 lengths: Pass one free end of strand from right to left hand. Simultaneously catch a loop around third finger of right hand. Make strands equal in thirds and cut the loops with scissors.

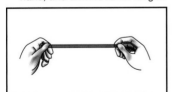

4. To make 1/4 lengths: Pass both free ends from right to left hand. Simultaneously catch a double loop around third finger of right hand. Cut the loops.

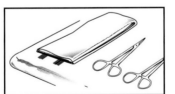

5. Place packets or strands in suture book (folded towel)–or under Mayo tray–with ends extended far enough to permit rapid extraction.

FIGURE 3.9 ... (From Ethicon Wound ..., Somerville, NJ, 2004, Ethicon.)

The surgeon places two hemostats on the vessel to be ligated and then cuts the vessel with Metzenbaum scissors or **electrocautery** (Fig. 3-10). Each end of the vessel is tied to maintain hemostasis. The sequence is as follows: clamp, clamp, cut, tie, and tie and cut suture material. The suture strand is tied around the vessel under the tip of the hemostat. The surgeon removes the hemostat after the first throw of the tie and then tightens the knot. Additional throws of the suture material secure the knot.

Larger vessels are often occluded with suture ligature or a **stick tie.** Stick ties are swaged on suture material with an **atraumatic** needle loaded on a needle driver. The most commonly used suture size for stick ties is 2-0 or 3-0.

Continuous ligature reels may be loaded with absorbable or nonabsorbable sutures and are usually used to occlude superficial bleeders. Regularly used reels contain chromic, plain, or Vicryl sutures. Ligature reels are **radiopaque** and considered a countable item in most facilities. The size of the suture material is specified by the number of holes on the top of the reel (Fig. 3-11).

Instrument Tie

The instrument tie is useful when one or both ends of a suture are short, and it has a variety of applications, particularly in facial surgery. Surgeon's knots and square knots are also used with the instrument tie. A *tie on a passer* or "instrument" tie is often used by the surgeon for deep bleeders not accessible with free ties. The surgeon may ask for a right angle for easier access to the vessel,

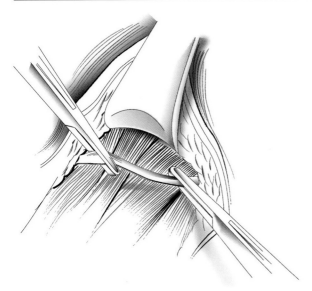

FIGURE **3-10** Drawing of two hemostats clamping a vessel. (From Ethicon: *Wound closure manual*, Somerville,

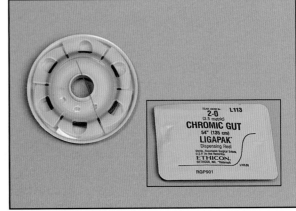

FIGURE **3-11** Suture reel.

followed by a needleless suture placed on a Schnidt tonsil clamp, hemostat, Adson, or Sarot clamp. The surgical technologist should have suture scissors available for the surgeon after the vessel is occluded.

Loading Sutures

The needle holder, or "needle driver," is the instrument used for placing sutures. It is the needle driver that pushes or drives the needle with the attached suture through tissue. The needle driver is held in the palm with the thumb and fourth finger (ring finger) in the rings of the handle (Fig. 3-12). The needle is grasped with the needle holder about two thirds from the pointed tip of the needle (Fig. 3-13). This helps to stabilize the needle and prevents it from bending.

Common Suture Techniques

The **primary suture line** is the line of sutures that holds the wound together during the healing process. It may be composed of a continuous strand of sutures or interrupted suture material. Specific uses for other types of sutures are deep sutures, buried sutures, purse-string sutures, and subcuticular sutures.

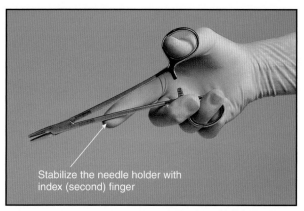

FIGURE **3-12** Needle driver held in the palm of the hand.

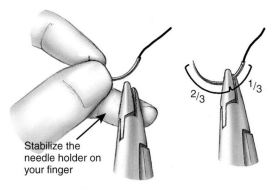

FIGURE **3-13** Loading the needle with the driver. (From Sherris DA, Kern EB: *Essential surgical skills,* ed 2, Philadelphia, 2004, Saunders.)

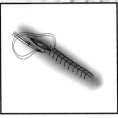

Looped suture, knotted at one end

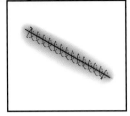

Two strands knotted at each end and knotted in the middle

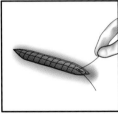

Running locked suture

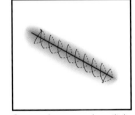

Over-and-over running stitch

FIGURE **3-14** Continuous suture line. (From Ethicon: *Wound closure manual*, Somerville, NJ, 2004, Ethicon.)

Continuous Sutures

Continuous sutures are also referred to as *running stitches*. A continuous suture has its strength evenly distributed along the entire suture line. The suture may be tied to itself at each end or looped with both cut ends of the suture tied together. Avoiding strangulation of tissues is important when suturing. Applying just firm tension instead of tight tension prevents any tissue damage. Continuous sutures allow for less foreign body mass in the wound. A continuous one-layer closure may be used on peritoneum or fascia layers of the abdominal wall, or both. The disadvantage of continuous suturing is that any suture breakage will disrupt the entire suture line (Fig. 3-14).

Interrupted Sutures

Interrupted sutures are placed separately in the wound. Each strand is tied and cut after suturing. An interrupted suture line provides a more secure closure because if one suture breaks, the remaining sutures hold the wound edges together until healing has occurred. Interrupted sutures are often used if a wound is infected because microorganisms are less able to travel along a series of interrupted sutures, thereby interrupting the pathway for bacteria.

Simple interrupted sutures are most commonly used. The sutures are positioned equally distant from each other (Fig. 3-15).

Vertical Mattress Sutures

Vertical mattress sutures require a two-bite suture method. The bites that are closer to the cut edge of the wound are used to accurately approximate and **evert** the skin edges (Fig. 3-16). This method is useful when the tissue has a tendency to **invert** with the placement of simple sutures.

Horizontal Mattress Sutures

Horizontal mattress sutures also require a two-bite suture method. The two bites are parallel to each other. Horizontal mattress sutures evert tissue but do not approximate tissue edges consistently. They may be used to take tension off the wound edge. This is followed with simple interrupted sutures or steri strips placed at the skin edge to precisely close the cut wound edges (Fig. 3-17).

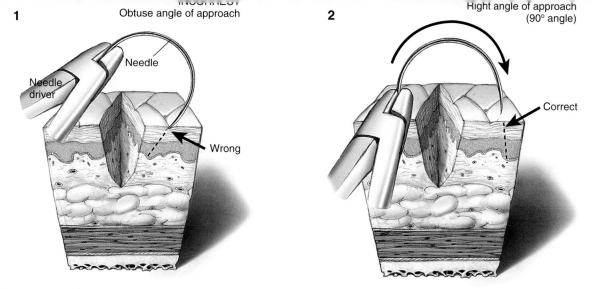

1

Needle

Needle driver

Wrong

2

Right angle of approach (90° angle)

Correct

FIGURE **3-15** Simple interrupted suture. (From Sherris DA, Kern EB: *Essential surgical skills,* ed 2, Philadelphia, 2004, Saunders.) *Continued*

3

Drive

4

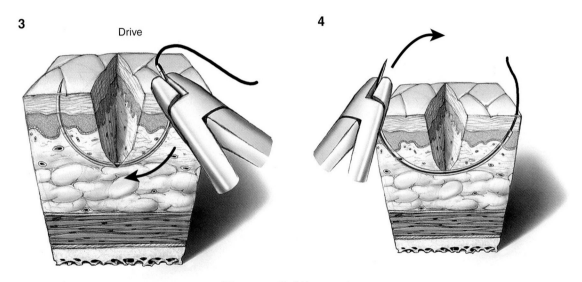

FIGURE **3-15** *Continued*

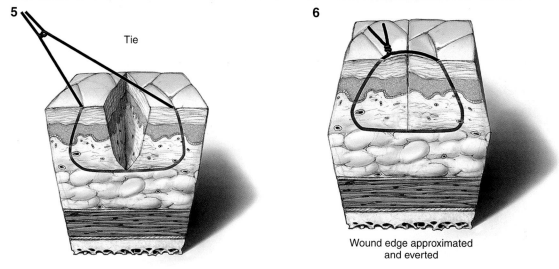

5

Tie

6

Wound edge approximated
and everted

FIGURE **3-15** *Continued*

Suture

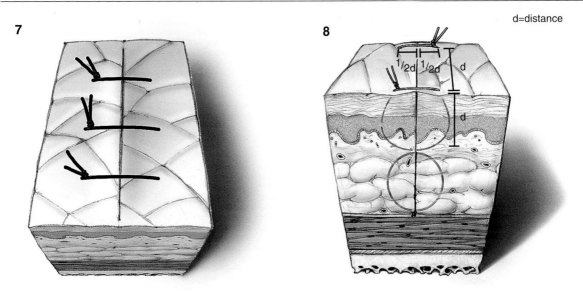

FIGURE **3-15** *Continued*

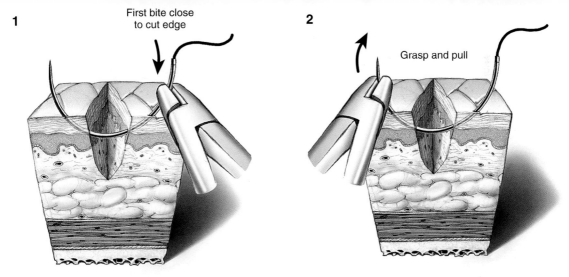

FIGURE **3-16** Interrupted vertical sutures. (From Sherris DA, Kern EB: *Essential surgical skills,* ed 2, Philadelphia, 2004, Saunders.)

Suture 68

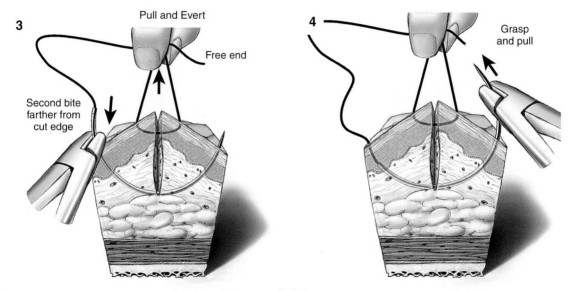

3 Pull and Evert

Free end

Second bite farther from cut edge

4 Grasp and pull

FIGURE **3-16** *Continued*

Continued

5

Tie

6

Vertical mattress

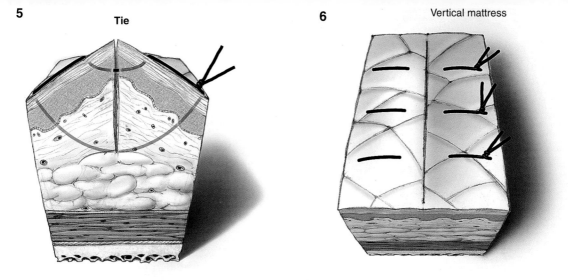

FIGURE **3-16** *Continued*

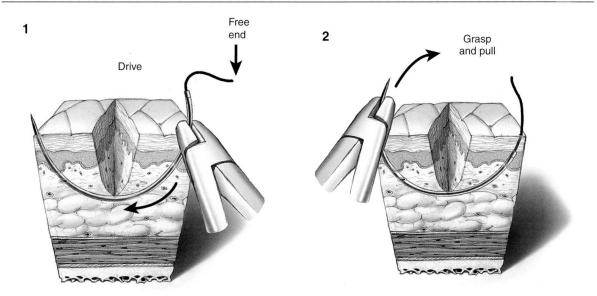

1 Drive

Free end

2 Grasp and pull

FIGURE **3-17** Horizontal mattress suture. (From Sherris DA, Kern EB: *Essential surgical skills,* ed 2, Philadelphia, 2004, Saunders.)

Continued

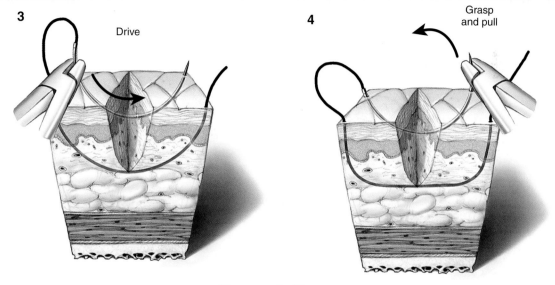

FIGURE **3-17** *Continued*

5   **Tie**

6   Horizontal mattress

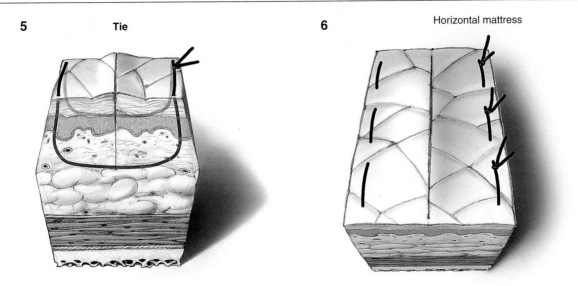

FIGURE **3-17** *Continued*

Running Closure (Baseball Stitch)

The running stitch is used when the wound's edges evert easily and a straight incision is being approximated. A running stitch should not be used if there is potential of hematomas, as all the sutures would have to be removed to drain the hematomas (Fig. 3-18).

Running Lock Closure

The running lock stitch is a deviation of the simple running closure or "baseball stitch." In the running lock, the stitch is locked before placement of the next stitch. This results in even more tissue eversion and less skin tension than a running stitch (Fig. 3-19).

Running Intracuticular Closure

A running **intracuticular** closure minimizes penetration of the skin with the needle. This closure is also described as subcuticular or running **intradermal** because it is placed in the dermis. This stitch is particularly useful for keloid patients where needle holes in the skin may encourage extreme scar formation. It is also practical for children as suture removal is fast and easy. No penetration of the epidermis exists except for the first and last bite of the stitch (Fig. 3-20).

1

2

Grasp and pull

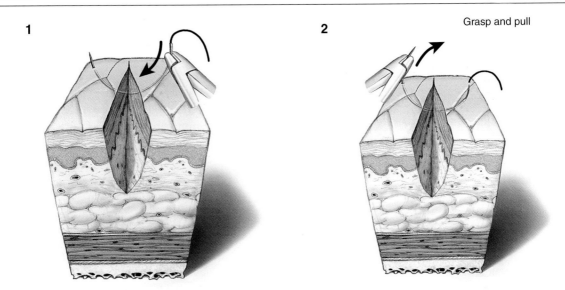

FIGURE **3-18** Running closure (baseball stitch). (From Sherris DA, Kern EB: *Essential surgical skills,* ed 2, Philadelphia, 2004, Saunders.)

Continued

3

Tie

4

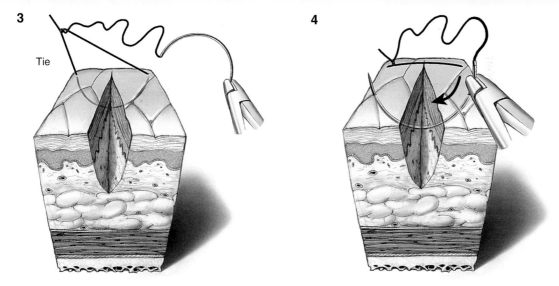

FIGURE **3-18** *Continued*

5

6

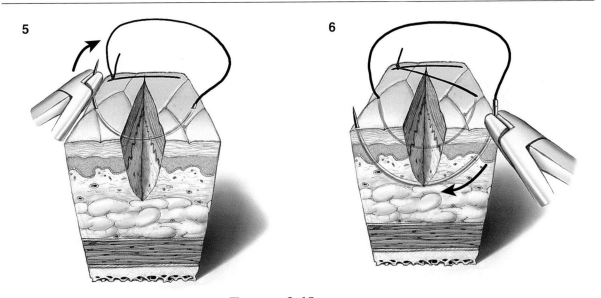

FIGURE **3-18** *Continued*

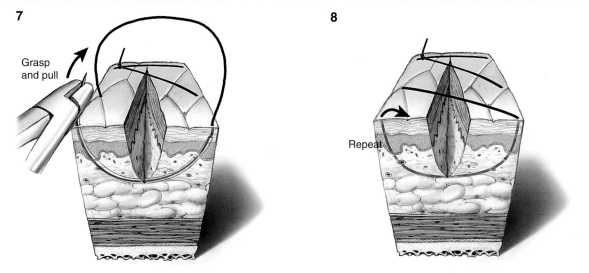

7

Grasp
and pull

8

Repeat

FIGURE **3-18** *Continued*

9

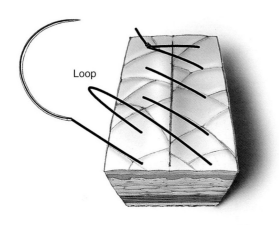

10

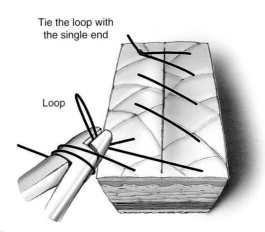

FIGURE **3-18** *Continued*

11

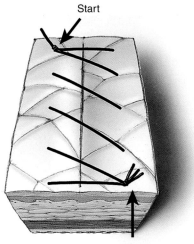

Start

Finish
(3 tails)

FIGURE **3-18** *Continued*

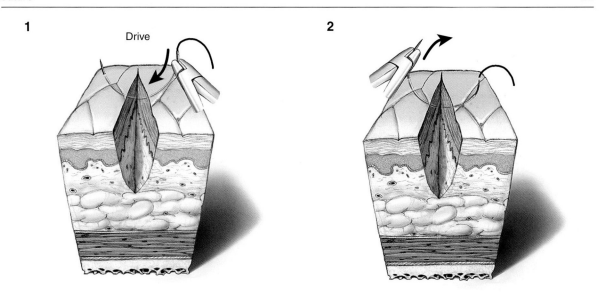

FIGURE **3-19** Running lock closure. (From Sherris DA, Kern EB: *Essential surgical skills,* ed 2, Philadelphia, 2004, Saunders.)

Continued

3

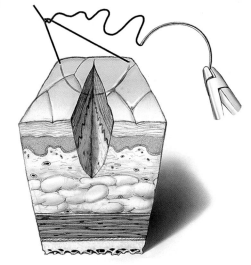

FIGURE **3-19** *Continued*

4

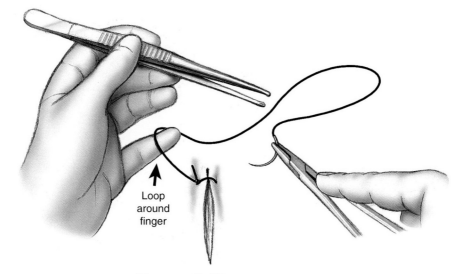

Loop around finger

FIGURE **3-19** *Continued*

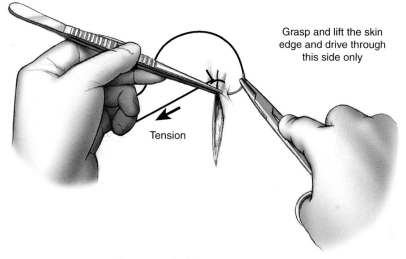

Grasp and lift the skin edge and drive through this side only

Tension

FIGURE **3-19** *Continued*

Suture

6

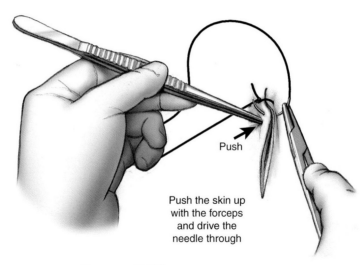

Push

Push the skin up
with the forceps
and drive the
needle through

FIGURE 3-19 *Continued*

7

Bring the loop down over the needle

8

Needle passes through the loop to lock

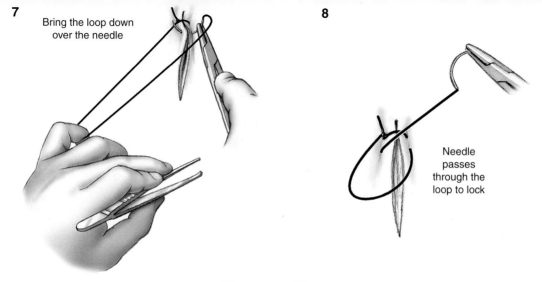

FIGURE **3-19** *Continued*

9

Repeat steps 4-8

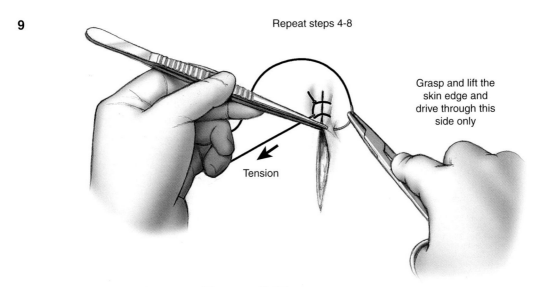

Grasp and lift the skin edge and drive through this side only

Tension

FIGURE **3-19** *Continued*

10

Wrap needle end
of suture around
needle driver,
grasp loop and
pull to tie

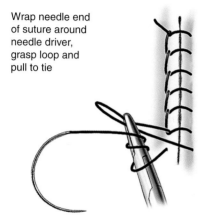

11

Running lock

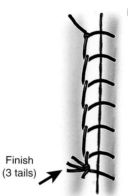

Finish
(3 tails)

FIGURE **3-19** *Continued*

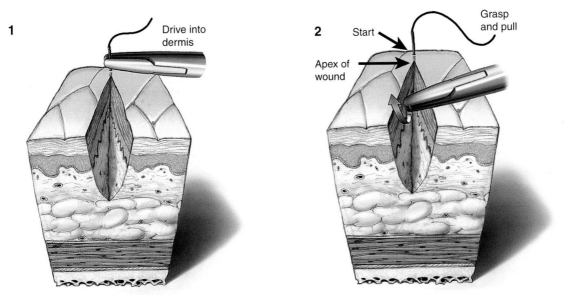

1 Drive into dermis

2 Start Apex of wound Grasp and pull

FIGURE **3-20** Running intracuticular closure. (From Sherris DA, Kern EB: *Essential surgical skills,* ed 2, Philadelphia, 2004, Saunders.)

Continued

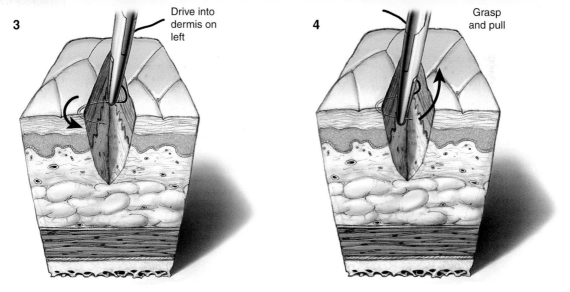

3 Drive into dermis on left

4 Grasp and pull

FIGURE **3-20** *Continued*

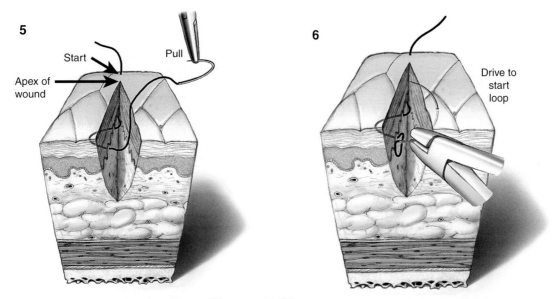

5 Start
Apex of wound
Pull

6 Drive to start loop

FIGURE **3-20** *Continued*

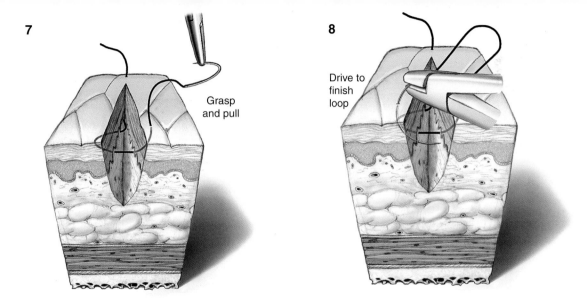

FIGURE **3-20** *Continued*

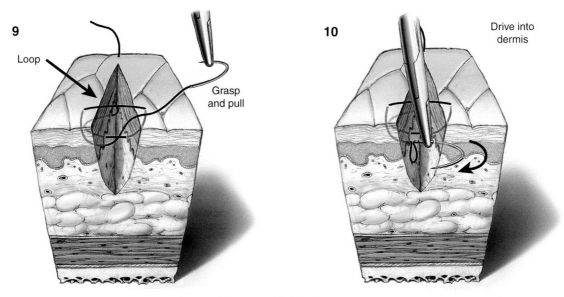

9

Loop

Grasp and pull

10

Drive into dermis

FIGURE **3-20** *Continued*

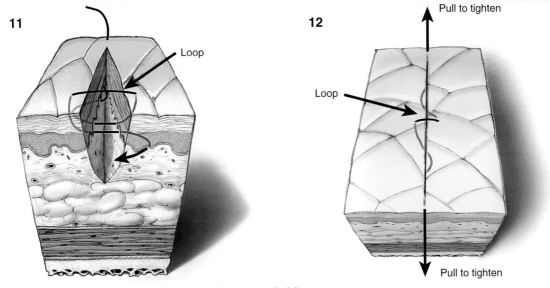

11

Loop

12

Pull to tighten

Loop

Pull to tighten

FIGURE **3-20** *Continued*

Deep Sutures

Deep sutures are completely buried under the epidermal skin layer. They may be continuous or interrupted sutures and are left as permanent sutures.

Buried Sutures

Buried sutures are positioned so that the knot protrudes to the inside, under the layer to be closed. This technique is often used with large-diameter permanent sutures placed in deeper layers in thin patients who may be able to feel large knots that are not buried (Fig. 3-21).

Purse-string Sutures

A drawstring suture placed in a circular motion around a lumen and then tightened to invert the opening is called a **purse-string suture**. Purse-string sutures are used around the stump of the appendix once the appendix is removed, in the bowel to secure an end-to-end anastomosis (EEA) stapling device, or in an organ such as the aorta to hold the cannulation tube in place during open heart surgery (Fig. 3-22).

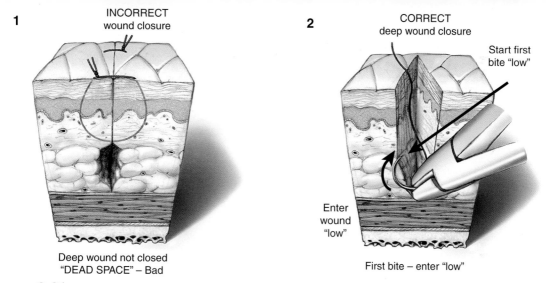

1 INCORRECT wound closure

Deep wound not closed "DEAD SPACE" – Bad

2 CORRECT deep wound closure

Start first bite "low"

Enter wound "low"

First bite – enter "low"

FIGURE **3-21** Buried sutures. (From Sherris DA, Kern EB: *Essential surgical skills,* ed 2, Philadelphia, 2004, Saunders.)
Continued

3

4

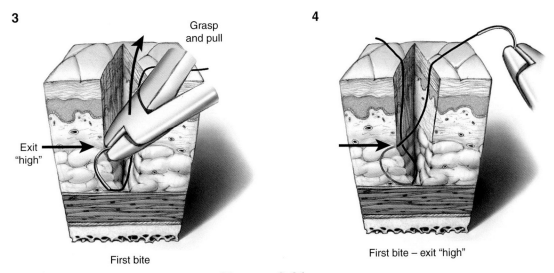

Grasp and pull

Exit "high"

First bite

First bite – exit "high"

FIGURE **3-21** *Continued*

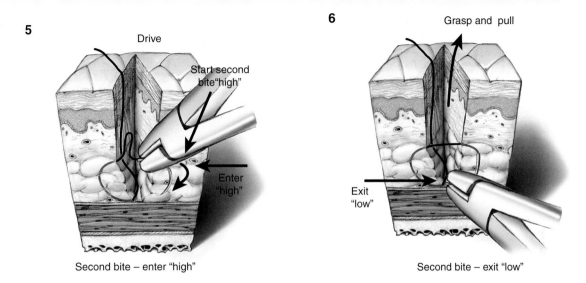

5

Drive

Start second
bite "high"

Enter
"high"

Second bite – enter "high"

6

Grasp and pull

Exit
"low"

Second bite – exit "low"

FIGURE **3-21** *Continued*

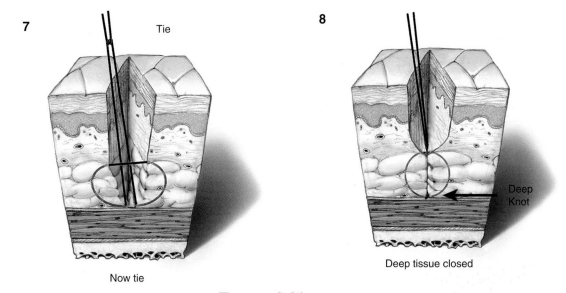

7 Tie

Now tie

8

Deep Knot

Deep tissue closed

FIGURE **3-21** *Continued*

9

Deep suture
cut on knot

10

Deep wound closed
with suture
No dead space

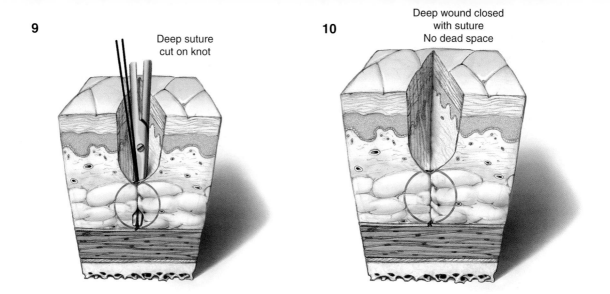

FIGURE **3-21** *Continued*

11

Drive

Skin closure

12

Wound closed correctly

Deep suture

Skin suture

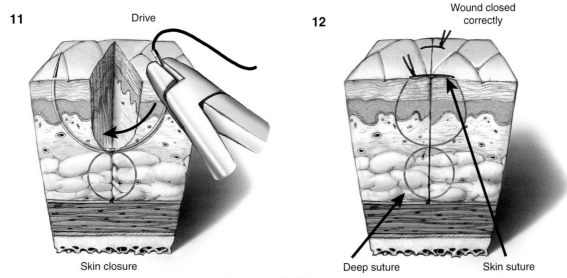

FIGURE **3-21** *Continued*

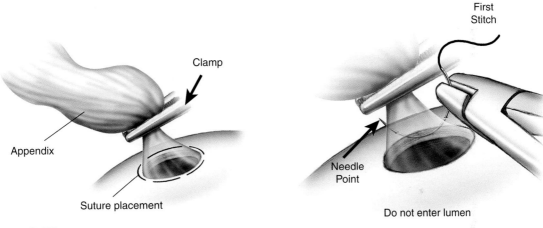

1

Clamp

Appendix

Suture placement

2

First Stitch

Needle Point

Do not enter lumen

FIGURE **3-22** Purse-string sutures. (From Sherris DA, Kern EB: *Essential surgical skills,* ed 2, Philadelphia, 2004, Saunders.)

Continued

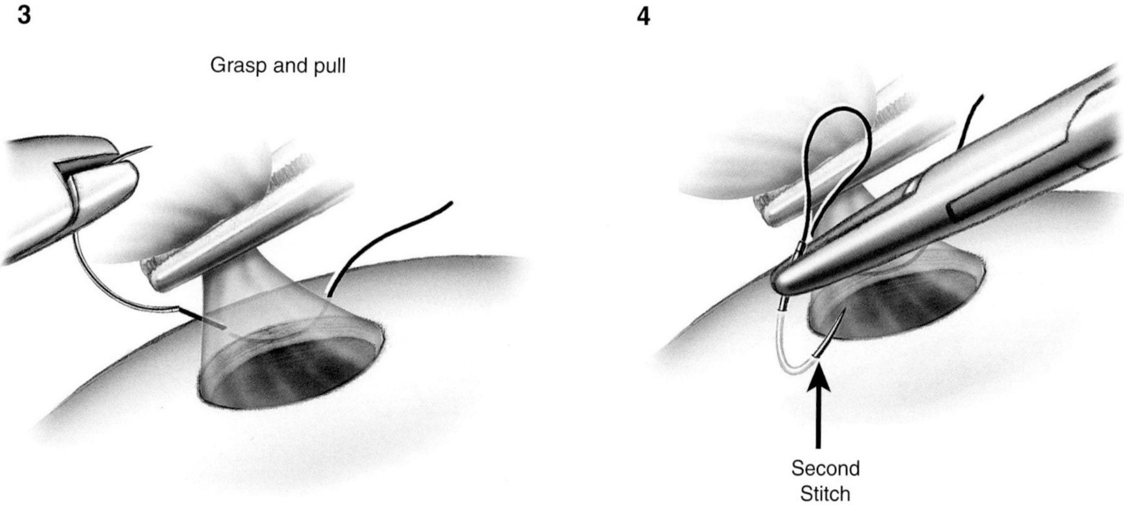

3

Grasp and pull

4

Second
Stitch

FIGURE **3-22** *Continued*

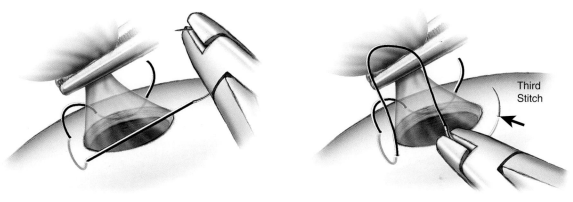

FIGURE **3-22** *Continued*

7

8

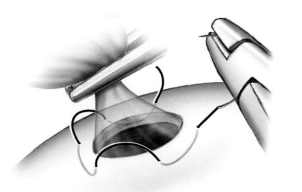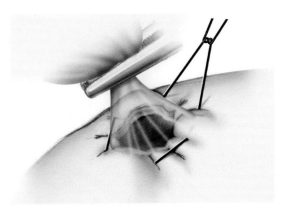

FIGURE **3-22** *Continued*

9

10

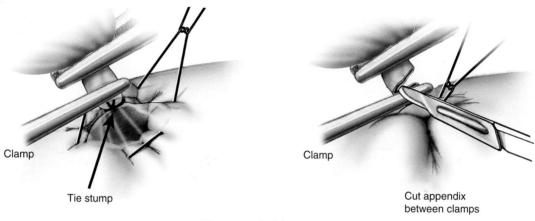

Clamp

Tie stump

Clamp

Cut appendix
between clamps

FIGURE **3-22** *Continued*

11   **12**

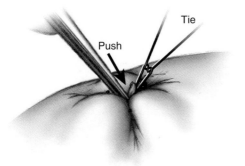

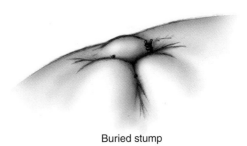

Buried stump

FIGURE **3-22** *Continued*

Subcuticular Sutures

The subcuticular stitch approximates the tough connective tissue just beneath the skin. A subcuticular stitch minimizes scarring. This technique involves short, lateral stitches the full length of the wound. Subcuticular sutures are continuous or interrupted sutures that are buried in the dermis, beneath the epithelial layer. Continuous subcuticular sutures are positioned in a line parallel to the wound. Subcuticular suturing is often performed with absorbable suture but may be placed with monofilament, nonabsorbable suture that is later removed.

Traction Sutures

Traction sutures may be used to retract tissue that is not easily held back with a conventional retractor. A nonabsorbable suture is placed into the structure, and the suture is then clamped with a hemostat. Tension on the suture retracts the tissue. Examples of places to use traction sutures are the myocardium of the heart, the sclera of the eye, and the tongue.

Secondary Suture Line

A secondary suture line is often used to support a primary suture line, eliminate dead space, or prevent fluid accumulation in an abdominal wound during healing by first intention (Fig. 3-23).

Retention Suture (Bolster) in Abdominal Wall

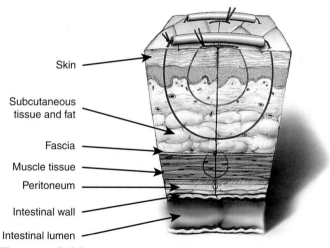

Skin

Subcutaneous
tissue and fat

Fascia

Muscle tissue

Peritoneum

Intestinal wall

Intestinal lumen

FIGURE 3-23 Secondary suture line. (From Sherris DA, Kern EB: *Essential surgical skills,* ed 2, Philadelphia, 2004, Saunders.)

Secondary suture lines also support wounds for healing by second intention, or a secondary closure following wound disruption when healing by third intention. Retention sutures are considered a secondary suture line.

Knot Construction
General Principles of Knot Tying

Although several hundred types of knots exist, only a few are used to ligate blood vessels or sutures. The type of knot used depends on the suture material selected, the depth and location of the incision, and the amount of stress to be placed on the wound postoperatively. If the knotted suture fails to carry out its function, the consequences could include massive bleeding. Wound dehiscence or an incisional hernia could also develop as a result. Each loop of suture that produces a knot is called a *throw*. Each throw can be either single or double.

The knot can be classified into two general types. The knot is considered a **square knot** if the "ear" and loop are parallel to each other and a **granny knot** if the right "ear" and loop cross different sides of the knot (Fig. 3-24). If the knot is constructed by an initial double-wrap throw followed by a single throw, it is considered a surgeon's knot.

Trauma to the suture by surgical instruments can seriously compromise suture efficacy. Grasping suture with clamps and forceps, as well as running one's fingers along the strand, could damage or weaken the suture material.

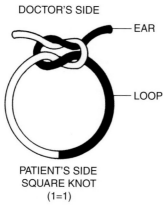

DOCTOR'S SIDE

EAR

LOOP

PATIENT'S SIDE
SQUARE KNOT
(1=1)

FIGURE 3-24 Components of a suture knot. (From Ethicon: *Wound closure manual,* Somerville, NJ, 2004, Ethicon.)

Principles of Knot Tying

The general principles of knot tying that apply to all suture material include the following:

- Ensure that the finished knot is firm enough to eliminate knot slippage.
- Tie the knot as small as possible and cut the ends as short as feasible. This prevents excessive tissue reaction toward absorbable sutures and minimizes foreign body reaction to nonabsorbable sutures.
- Avoid damaging the suture material when handling.
- Avoid excessive tension, which may cause sutures to break and cut tissue.
- Be careful to not tie sutures too tightly when approximating tissue, as this may lead to tissue strangulation. Remember: **Approximate—do not strangulate!**
- Sustain traction at one end of the suture once the first loop is tied to prevent loosening of the throw.

GRANNY KNOT TYPE

Granny Knot 1x1

Surgeon's Knot
Granny 2x1

Reverse Surgeon's
Knot Granny 1x2

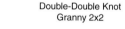

Double-Double Knot
Granny 2x2

SQUARE KNOT TYPE

Square Knot 1x1

Surgeon's Knot
Square 2x1

Reverse Surgeon's
Knot Square 1x2

Double-Double Knot
Square 2x2

FIGURE **3-25** Square knot. (From Ethicon: *Wound closure manual,* Somerville, NJ, 2004, Ethicon.)

- Remember that a seesaw motion over the suture when forming a knot will cause it to break down.
- Ensure that the final throw is as horizontal as possible.
- Remember that extra throws of the suture only add bulk to the knot; they do not strengthen it.

Square Knot

The two-handed **square knot** is the most reliable type of knot and easiest to learn. It is also the most useful. The square knot, as well as the surgeon's knot, is considered complete after three to six throws, depending on the suture material used and the surgeon's ability. Braided suture is easier to tie and holds a knot more securely. For example, silk suture will hold a knot after three to four throws, while Prolene is secure after five to seven throws (Fig. 3-25). This is to ensure a knot is secure.

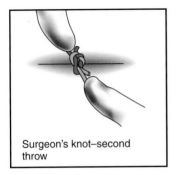

Surgeon's knot–second throw

FIGURE **3-26** Surgeon's knot. (From Ethicon: *Wound closure manual,* Somerville, NJ, 2004, Ethicon.)

Surgeon's Knot

The difference between the square knot and the surgeon's knot is that the square knot has one loop in the first throw and the surgeon's knot has two loops. Once the first loop is completed, the knot construction is the same. Subsequent throws are always opposite of the previous throw to improve the security of the tie. The surgeon's knot is more secure than the square knot with the extra loop before the second throw (Fig. 3-26).

Figure-of-Eight Stick Tie

The figure-of-eight stick tie is a variation of the free vessel ligature and is indicated for larger vessels of tissue pedicles. The stick tie is less likely to become loosened or fall off during the postoperative period. The first throw is the surgeon's knot. The free ends are then passed around the two sides of the instrument clamp, and the knot is completed with subsequent throws (Fig. 3-27).

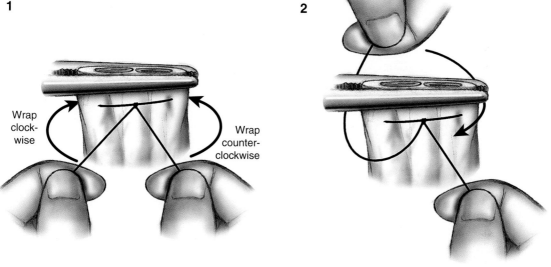

1

Wrap clock-wise

Wrap counter-clockwise

2

FIGURE **3-27** Figure-of-eight stick tie. (From Sherris DA, Kern EB: *Essential surgical skills,* ed 2, Philadelphia, 2004, Saunders.)

Continued

3

4

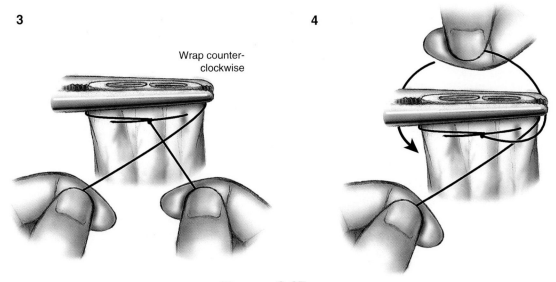

Wrap counter-clockwise

FIGURE **3-27** *Continued*

5

Assistant releases hemostat slowly
while surgeon ties

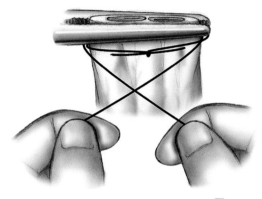

6

Hemostasis secured

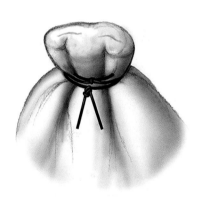

FIGURE **3-27** *Continued*

Anatomy of Surgical Needles

The main purpose of the surgical needle is to penetrate the wound edges so that sutures can approximate the tissue and close the wound. The main considerations for needle selection are (1) the type of tissue being closed; and (2) curvature of the needle, which is based on the space of the operative field. Needle sharpness and **ductility** (the needle's resistance to breaking and bending when it enters tissue) are important factors when selecting a needle.

Surgical needles are produced from stainless steel alloys, which have excellent resistance to corrosion. Since the advancement of surgical needles in the 1960s, high nickel **maraging** stainless steel has been used extensively due to the greater resistance to bending and breakage than stainless steels without nickel. A high nickel maraging stainless steel is composed of 7.5% to 9.5% nickel, along with titanium and chromium. SURGALLOY, a high nickel stainless steel, is currently used to manufacture surgical needles. Every surgical needle has three basic components: swage, body, and point (Fig. 3-28).

Needle size is measured in inches or metric units. Several dimensions determine the size of the needle (Fig. 3-29):

- Chord length—the straight-line distance from the point of a curved needle to the swage
- Needle length—the distance measured along the needle itself from point to end
- Radius—the distance from the center of the circle to the body of the needle if the curvature of the needle were continued to make a full circle
- Diameter—the gauge or thickness of the needle wire

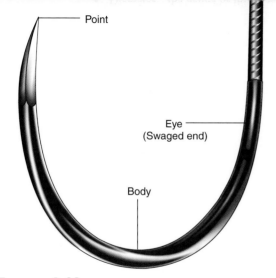

FIGURE **3-28** Needle components. (From Ethicon: *Wound closure manual,* Somerville, NJ, 2004, Ethicon.)

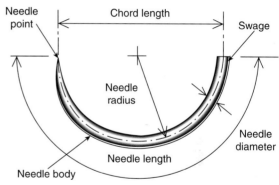

FIGURE **3-29** Anatomy of a needle. (From Ethicon: *Wound closure manual,* Somerville, NJ, 2004, Ethicon.)

Suture

Before 1914, needles used by surgeons were compatible to sewing needles, with eyes at the end for holding suture. The eye's diameter was wider than the rest of the needle. Needles needed to be hand threaded. The eye is separated into one of three categories: closed eye, French eye, or swaged (eyeless) (Fig. 3-30).

Because swaged needles are less traumatic to tissue, nearly all surgical needles today are swaged. When the surgeon is finished placing suture in the tissue, the suture may be cut or released from the needle, such in the case of a control-release needle.

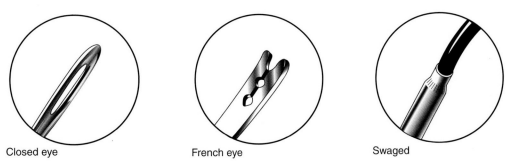

Closed eye   French eye   Swaged

FIGURE 3-30 Closed eye, French eye, and swaged eye. (From Ethicon: *Wound closure manual,* Somerville, NJ, 2004, Ethicon.)

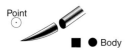

FIGURE **3-31** Tapered needle. (From Ethicon: *Wound closure manual,* Somerville, NJ, 2004, Ethicon.)

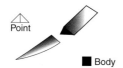

FIGURE **3-32** Cutting needle. (From Ethicon: *Wound closure manual,* Somerville, NJ, 2004, Ethicon.)

Common Needle Types

The most commonly used needles in surgery today include cutting and tapered (Fig. 3-31). The tapered needle minimizes tissue trauma because the needle pierces tissue without cutting it. The needle point tapers to a sharp tip and then flattens to an oval or rectangle shape. Tapered-point needles are also referred to as *round needles.* They are mostly used in general surgery for closure of the peritoneum, abdominal viscera, myocardium, dura, and subcutaneous layers.

The cutting needle has at least two opposing cutting edges (Fig. 3-32). They are designed to cut through tough, difficult-to-penetrate tissue. Cutting needles are ideal for skin sutures that pass through dense, irregular, and relatively thick connective dermal tissue. Special plastic surgery needles are perfect for delicate facial surgery because they have a narrow point with a thin taper, allowing soft tissue to be easily penetrated.

Reverse cutting, or "cutting," needles are designed with the cutting edge on the outer convex side. Reverse cutting needles were designed to pierce tough tissue without bending or breaking the needle (Fig. 3-33). This includes skin, oral mucosa, tendon sheaths,

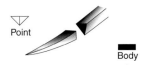

FIGURE **3-33** Reverse cutting needle.
(From Ethicon: *Wound closure manual,*
Somerville, NJ, 2004, Ethicon.)

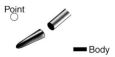

FIGURE **3-34** Blunt-tip needle. (From
Ethicon: *Wound closure manual,* Somerville,
NJ, 2004, Ethicon.)

periosteum, and other tough tissue. Reverse cutting is also excellent for cosmetic, ophthalmic surgery because of the minimal tissue trauma and minimal scar formation.

Blunt point needles dissect friable tissue rather than cutting through it. They have a tapered body with a rounded, blunt point that does not cut tissue. Blunt point needles are used for suturing the liver and kidneys. Due to safety considerations, surgeons also use blunt point needles in obstetric and gynecologic procedures. Blunt-tip needles are effective in procedures on high-risk patients (Fig. 3-34).

The DermaX needle by Syneture contains four cutting edges with a double point tip. It is designed to move smoothly with precision control through subcuticular/cuticular tissues of body structures like the forehead, eyelids, nose, chin, and breast (Fig. 3-35).

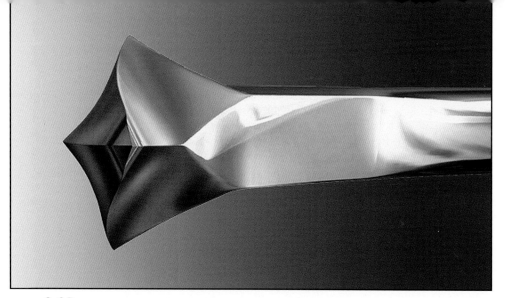

FIGURE **3-35** DermaX needle. (Courtesy United States Surgical, a division of Tyco Healthcare Group LP.)

Suture

Suture Material

CHAPTER 4

Twisted, Absorbable Suture Material
Natural
Plain Gut

Plain gut is composed of collagen material prepared from the submucosal layers of the small intestine of healthy sheep or the serosal layers of the small intestines of healthy cattle. It is characterized by the following (Fig. 4-1):

- Indicated for use in general soft tissue approximation or ligation
- 5-10 day wound support and an absorption rate of 30-60 days
- Dissolved by enzymes
- Contraindicated in cardiovascular and neurologic tissue
- Inappropriate for use in elderly, malnourished, or debilitated patients
- Available in precut lengths, ligating reels, or free ties
- Supplied in sizes 7-0 through 3 (0.7 to 7) and 0 through 1 (metric 4 to 5) in control release

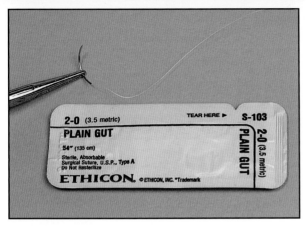

FIGURE 4-1 Plain gut. (Courtesy Ethicon, 2004, Somerville, NJ.)

- Advantages: produces only minimal tissue reaction during absorption
- Disadvantages: wound dehiscence, failure to provide wound support

Fast Absorbing Gut Suture Material

Fast absorbing gut suture is composed of collagen material prepared from the submucosal layers of the small intestine of healthy sheep or the serosal layers of the small intestines of healthy cattle. It is characterized by the following (Fig. 4-2):

- Indicated for use on dermal (skin) suturing only
- 5-7 day wound support and an absorption rate of 20 to 40 days
- Heat treated to break down quicker
- Undyed
- Dissolved by enzymes
- Contraindicated for internal tissue
- Inappropriate for use in elderly, malnourished, or debilitated patients

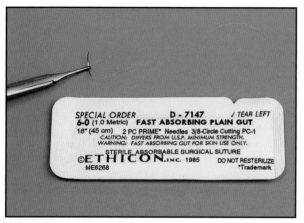

FIGURE **4-2** Fast absorbing gut. (Courtesy Ethicon, 2004, Somerville, NJ.)

- Available in precut lengths 5-0 (metric 1.5) and 6-0 (metric 1)
- Advantages: Produces only minimal tissue reaction during absorption
- Disadvantages: wound dehiscence, failure to provide wound support

Chromic Gut Suture Material

Chromic gut suture is composed of collagen material prepared from the submucosal layers of the small intestine of healthy sheep or the serosal layers of the small intestines of healthy cattle. It is coated with chromic salts and is characterized by the following (Fig. 4-3, *A* through *C*):

- 10-14 day wound support and an absorption rate of 60 to 90 days
- Processed to provide greater resistance to absorption
- Dissolved by enzymatic process
- Suture contains memory
- Often used in gynecologic procedures
- Suture is dyed tan or beige

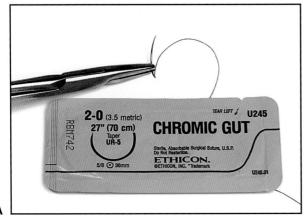
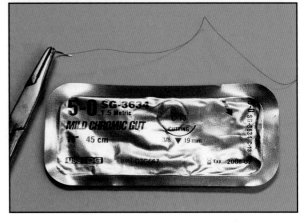

FIGURE **4-3** Chromic suture. (Courtesy Ethicon, 2004, Somerville, NJ. Reprinted from United States Surgical, a division of Tyco Healthcare Group, LP.) *Continued*

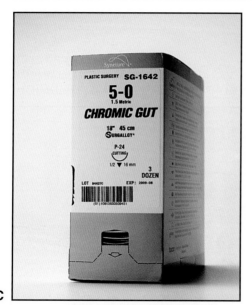

C

FIGURE **4-3** *Continued*

- Inappropriate for use in elderly, malnourished, or debilitated patients
- Available in precut lengths, ligating reels, or free ties
- Supplied in sizes 7-0 through 3 (0.7 to 7) and 0 through 1 (metric 4 to 5) in control release
- Advantages: produces less tissue reaction because of salt coating
- Disadvantages: wound dehiscence, failure to provide wound support

Monofilament Absorbable Suture Material Synthetic

Monocryl: Poliglecaprone 25

Monocryl suture material is prepared from a copolymer of glycolide and epsilon-caprolactone. Poliglecaprone 25 copolymer has been found to be nonantigenic and nonpyrogenic and elicits only a slight tissue reaction during absorption. It is characterized by the following (Fig. 4-4):

- 14-day wound support and an absorption rate of 91 to 119 days with greater tensile strength than chromic gut suture
- Indicated for use in general soft tissue approximation

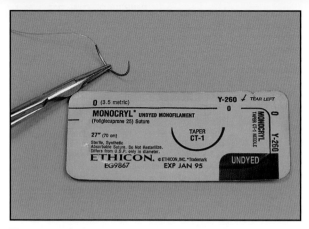

FIGURE **4-4** Monocryl suture. (Courtesy Ethicon, 2004, Somerville, NJ.)

- Not indicated for use in cardiovascular or neurologic tissues, microsurgery, or ophthalmic surgery
- Available in violet dyed or undyed suture (the latter of which is used in skin sutures)
- Available in precut lengths of 6-0 through 2 (metric sizes 0 to 7.5)
- Available in 3-0 through 1 (metric sizes 2-4) attached to control release
- Swaged needles and control release suture
- Advantages: minimal reaction in tissues
- Disadvantages: may be treated as a foreign body

Caprosyn Suture: Polyglytone 6211

Caprosyn suture material is a synthetic polyester composed of glycolide, caprolactone, trimethylene carbonate, and lactide. It is characterized by the following (Fig. 4-5, *A* through *C*):

- 10-day wound support and a maximum absorption rate of 56 days
- Indicated for use in general soft tissue approximation

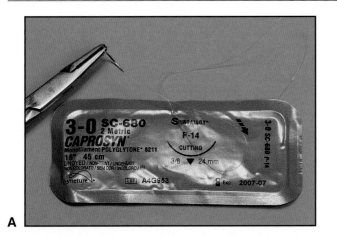

FIGURE **4-5** Caprosyn suture. (Courtesy United States Surgical, a division of Tyco Healthcare Group, LP.)

Continued

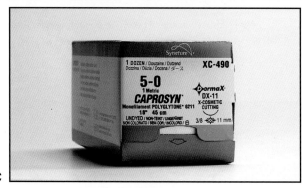

C

FIGURE 4-5 *Continued*

- Not indicated for use in cardiovascular or neurologic tissues, microsurgery, or ophthalmic surgery
- Available in violet dyed or undyed suture (the latter of which is used in skin suture)
- Often used in skin closures
- Available in precut lengths of 6-0 through 2 (metric sizes 0 to 7.5)
- Available in 3-0 through 1 (metric sizes 2-4) attached to control release
- Swaged needles and control release suture
- Advantages: minimal reaction in tissues
- Disadvantages: risk of wound dehiscence

Biosyn Suture Material: Glycomer 631

Biosyn suture material is a synthetic polyester composed of glycolide (60%), dioxanone (14%), and trimethylene carbonate (26%). It is characterized by the following (Fig. 4-6, *A* and *B*):
- 21-day wound support and an absorption rate of 90 to 110 days
- Absorbed by hydrolysis

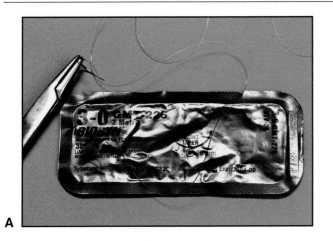

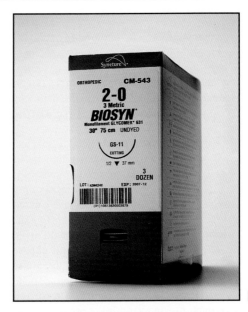

FIGURE **4-6** Biosyn suture. (Courtesy United States Surgical, a division of Tyco Healthcare Group, LP.)

- Indicated for use in general soft tissue approximation or ligation, or both, including use in ophthalmic surgery
- Suture is available undyed or violet
- Inappropriate for use in cardiovascular or neurologic surgery
- Contraindicated when extended approximation of tissue is required
- Available in precut lengths and ligapak reels
- Disadvantages: wound dehiscence, failure to provide wound support

Maxon Suture Material: Polyglyconate

Maxon suture material is prepared from a copolymer of glycolic acid and trimethylene carbonate. It is characterized by the following (Fig. 4-7, *A* and *B*):
- 6-week wound support and an absorption rate of 6 months
- Maxon is indicated for soft tissue approximation or ligation, or both
- Indicated for use in pediatric cardiovascular and peripheral vascular tissue
- Maxon and Maxon CV are not indicated for use in adult cardiovascular tissue, ophthalmic surgery, microsurgery, and neural tissue
- Available in precut lengths, ligating reels, free ties
- Maxon is available in sizes 1 through 7-0
- Maxon CV is available in U.S. Pharmacopeia (USP) sizes 7-0 through 4-0
- Maxon sutures are available green or undyed

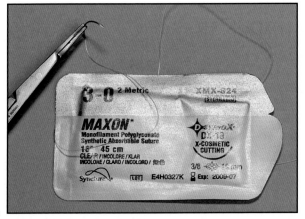

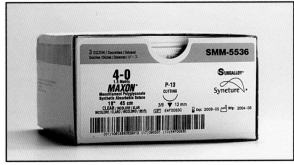

FIGURE **4-7** Maxon/Maxon CV suture. (Courtesy United States Surgical, a division of Tyco Healthcare Group, LP.)

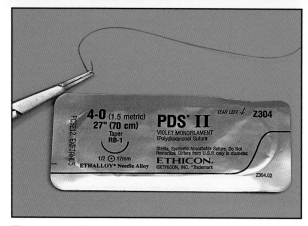

FIGURE **4-8** PDS II suture. (Courtesy Ethicon, 2004, Somerville, NJ.)

- Disadvantages: wound dehiscence or delayed wound healing if expansion, stretching or distension occurs

PDS II Suture Material: Polydioxanone

PDS II suture material is synthetic fiber produced from petroleum byproducts. It is characterized by the following (Fig. 4-8):

- 6-week wound support and an absorption rate of 6 months
- Indicated for use in soft tissue approximation including pediatric cardiovascular tissue, where growth is expected, and ophthalmic surgery
- PDS II is not indicated for use in adult cardiovascular tissue, microsurgery, and neural tissue
- Available in precut lengths, ligating reels, and free ties
- PDS II is available in violet dyed sizes of 2 through 9-0 (metric size 0.3 to 5) and blue dyed strands in sizes 9-0 through 7-0 (metric sizes 0.3-0.5) in various lengths

- PDS II violet suture is available in USP sizes 4-0 through 1 (metric sizes 0.5-4) in control release
- Clear sutures are available in sizes 7-0 through 1 (metric size 0.5-4) with permanently attached needles
- Contraindicated with prosthetic devices (i.e., heart valves or synthetic grafts)

Monodek (Deknatel)

Monodek (Deknatel) suture material is characterized by the following:
- 2-week wound support and an absorption rate of 14 to 21 days
- Absorbed by hydrolysis
- Indicated for use in plastic and reconstructive, cosmetic, ophthalmic, pediatric cardiovascular, and general surgical procedures
- Has a low risk for wicking
- Available in precut lengths and ligapak reels
- Monodek is offered in sizes 6-0 through 0 (metric sizes 0.7 to 3.5)

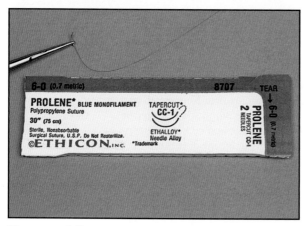

FIGURE **4-9** Prolene suture. (Courtesy Ethicon, 2004, Somerville, NJ.)

Prolene Suture Material: Polypropylene

Prolene suture material is composed of isotactic crystalline stereoisomer of polypropylene, a synthetic linear polyolefin. The suture material, which may be dyed blue to enhance visibility, is characterized by the following (Fig. 4-9):

- Encapsulated in tissue
- Indicated for use in soft tissue approximation including cardiovascular, ophthalmic, and neurologic procedures
- Available in precut lengths, ligating reels, and free ties
- Easily damaged or crushed by instruments
- Prolene suture is available in USP sizes 4-0 through 1 (metric sizes 0.5-4) in control release
- Clear sutures are available in sizes 7-0 through 1 (metric size 0.5-4) with permanently attached needles
- One of the most inert sutures available
- Very useful in the presence of infection and for vascular anastomosis

Surgipro II Suture Material: Polypropylene

Surgipro II suture material is composed of isotactic crystalline stereoisomer of polypropylene, a synthetic linear polyolefin. The suture material, which is clear or pigmented blue to enhance visibility, is characterized by the following (Fig. 4-10, *A* and *B*):

- Encapsulated in tissue
- Indicated for use in soft tissue approximation including cardiovascular, ophthalmic, and neurologic procedures
- Available in precut lengths, ligating reels, and free ties
- Easily damaged or crushed by instruments
- Surgipro suture is available in USP sizes 10-0 through 2 (metric sizes 0.2-5) in control release
- Surgipro II is available in sizes 8-0 through 3-0 (0.4-2 metric)
- Also available in polytetrafluoroethylene (PTFE) pledgets or bead and collar components to anchor the ends of the suture for subcuticular closure or use in tendon sutures
- One of the most inert sutures available
- Useful in the presence of infection and for vascular anastomosis

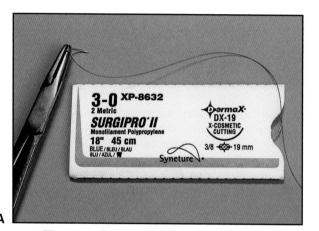
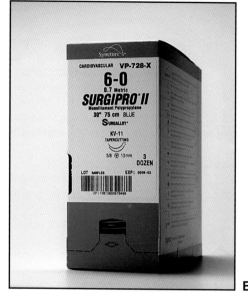

FIGURE **4-10** Surgipro. (Courtesy United States Surgical, a division of Tyco Healthcare Group, LP.)

Deklene Suture Material: Polypropylene

Deklene suture material is composed of isotactic crystalline stereoisomer of polypropylene, a synthetic linear polyolefin. This monofilament suture is clear or pigmented blue to enhance visibility. It is characterized by the following:

- Suture is encapsulated in tissue
- Uniform diameter with high tensile strength and resists breaking
- Easily damaged or crushed by instruments
- Deklene suture is available in USP sizes 9-0 through 2 (metric sizes 0.3 to 5) in control release
- Useful in the presence of infection and for vascular anastomosis

Novafil Suture Material: Polybutester

Novafil suture material is composed of copolymer of butylene terephthalate and polytetramethylene ether glycol. The suture material is clear or pigmented with copper phthalocyanine blue. It is characterized by the following (Fig. 4-11, *A* and *B*):

- Encapsulated in tissue
- Indicated for use in soft tissue approximation including cardiovascular and ophthalmic
- Contraindicated in microsurgery or neurologic procedures
- Available in precut lengths, ligating reels, and free ties
- Easily damaged or crushed by instruments

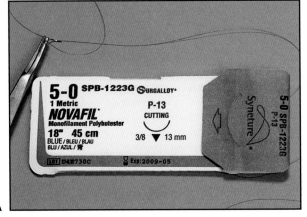
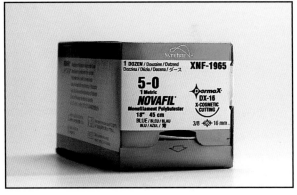

FIGURE **4-11** Novafil suture. (Courtesy United States Surgical, a division of Tyco Healthcare Group, LP.)

- Novafil suture is available in USP sizes 2 through 10-0 (metric sizes 0.2 to 5) and in control release
- Adequate knot security requires the technique of flat, square ties
- Low tissue reaction

Vascufil Suture Material: Polybutester

Vascufil suture material is composed of copolymer of butylene terephthalate and polytetramethylene ether glycol. The suture material is coated with polytribolate, an absorbable polymer of e-caprolactone/glycolide/poloxamer 188. It is characterized by the following (Fig. 4-12, *A* and *B*):

- Encapsulated in tissue
- Indicated for use in soft tissue approximation including cardiovascular and ophthalmic
- Contraindicated in microsurgery or neurologic procedures. Also not recommended for patients suffering from cancer, anemia, obesity, diabetes, infections, or any conditions that delay wound healing
- Available in precut lengths and free ties
- Disadvantages: wound dehiscence; failure to provide wound support in closure sites of expansion, stretching, or where distension occurs

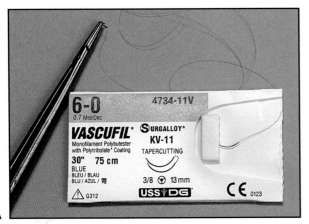

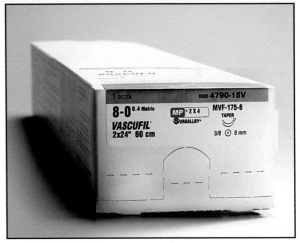

FIGURE **4-12** Vascufil suture. (Courtesy United States Surgical, a division of Tyco Healthcare Group, LP.)

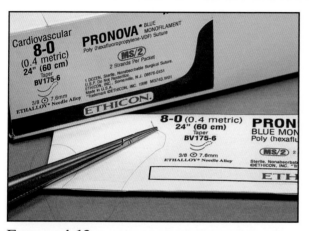

FIGURE **4-13** Pronova suture. (Courtesy Ethicon, 2004, Somerville, NJ.)

Pronova Suture Material: Poly (Hexafluoropropylene-VDF)

Pronova suture material is a nonabsorbable, sterile surgical suture made from a polymer blend of poly (vinylidene fluoride) and poly (vinylidene fluoride-co-hexafluoropropylene). The suture material is pigmented blue to enhance visibility, except for 7-0, which is clear. It is characterized by the following (Fig. 4-13):

- Encapsulated in tissue
- Indicated for use in soft tissue approximation including cardiovascular and ophthalmic
- No known contraindications
- Available in precut lengths and free ties
- Pronova suture is available in USP sizes 10-0 through 8-0 (metric sizes 0.2 to 0.4)
- Disadvantages: wound dehiscence, calculi formation in urinary and biliary tracts when prolonged contact with salt solutions

Ethilon Suture Material: Nylon

Ethilon suture material is composed of the long chain aliphatic polymers Nylon 6 and Nylon 6.6. Ethilon sutures are dyed black or green to enhance visibility in tissue. They are also available in clear. This suture material is characterized by the following:

- Suture is encapsulated in tissue
- Indicated for use in soft tissue approximation including cardiovascular and ophthalmic
- Available in precut lengths and free ties
- Disadvantages: wound dehiscence, failure to provide wound support in closure sites of expansion, stretching, or where distension occurs
- Produced in sizes 11-0 through 2 (metric sizes 0.1 to 5)

Dermalon Suture Material: Nylon

Dermalon suture material is composed of the long chain aliphatic polymers Nylon 6 and Nylon 6.6. Dermalon are coated uniformly with silicone to enhance handling and passage through the tissue. Sutures are dyed black or blue to enhance visibility in tissue. Clear sutures are also available. Dermalon suture material is characterized by the following (Fig. 4-14, *A* and *B*):

- Encapsulated in tissue
- Indicated for use in soft tissue approximation including cardiovascular and ophthalmic
- Available in precut lengths, ligating reels, and free ties

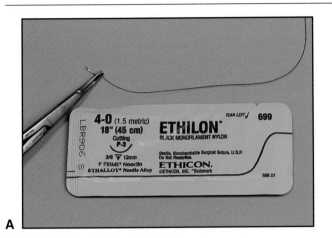

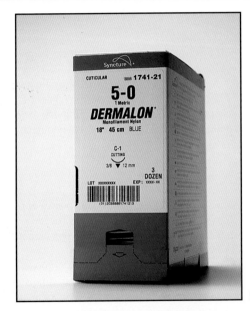

FIGURE **4-14** Ethilon/Dermalon. (Courtesy Ethicon, 2004, Somerville, NJ. Reprinted from United States Surgical, a division of Tyco Healthcare Group, LP.)

- Disadvantages: wound dehiscence; failure to support wound in closure sites of expansion, stretching, or where distension occurs
- Produced in sizes 6-0 through 1 (metric sizes 0.1 to 4)

Monosof Suture Material: Nylon

Monosof suture material is composed of the long chain aliphatic polymers Nylon 6 and Nylon 6.6. Monosof sutures are coated uniformly with silicone to enhance handling and passage through the tissue. Sutures are dyed black or clear and are characterized by the following (Fig. 4-15, *A* and *B*):
- Encapsulated in tissue
- Indicated for use in soft tissue approximation including cardiovascular and ophthalmic tissue
- Available in precut lengths, ligating reels, and free ties
- Disadvantages: wound dehiscence, knot slippage
- Produced in sizes 7-0 through 0 (metric sizes 0.1 to 4)

Force Fiber (Deknatel): Polyethylene

Teleflex Medical Force Fiber is a nonabsorbable surgical suture composed of high-molecular-weight polyethylene fiber. It is characterized by the following:
- The Force Fiber suture contains Dyneema Purity, a material fiber for high performance applications.
- Dyneema Purity is 15 times stronger than steel.
- Force Fiber suture has flexibility; pliability; and a nonabrasive, silklike touch.

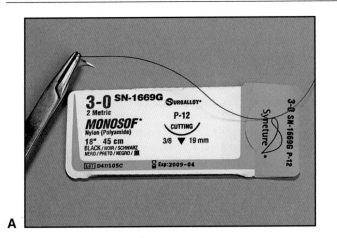

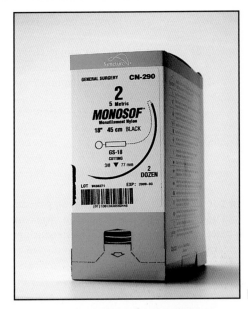

FIGURE **4-15** Monosof suture. (Courtesy United States Surgical. Reprinted from United States Surgical, a division of Tyco Healthcare Group, LP.)

Monofilament or Multifilament Nonabsorbable Suture Material
Synthetic
Steel Suture Material: Stainless Steel

Steel suture material is composed of 316L stainless steel conforming to American Society for Testing and Materials (ASTM) Standard F138 grade 2 "stainless steel bar and wire for surgical implants." Steel sutures meet all requirements established by the USP and are characterized by the following:

- Encapsulated in tissue
- Indicated for use in abdominal wound closure, intestinal anastomosis, hernia repair, sternal closure, and some orthopedic procedures (e.g., cerclage, tendon repair)
- Available in precut lengths, nonneedled or affixed to needles with permanent needle attachment techniques or ROTOGRIP
- Contraindicated in patients with known sensitivities or allergies to steel and its principal metallic components, chromium and nickel; additionally, the presence of steel may interfere with certain radiodiagnostics and its use is contraindicated where radiotransparency of suture is required
- Available in monofilament sizes 6-0 through 7 (metric sizes 0.7 to 9)

Table 4-1 Stainless Steel Suture Comparison

Size (USP)	B & S Gauge	Size (USP)	B & S Gauge
6-0	40	0	26
6-0	38	1	25
5-0	35	2	24
4-0	34	3	23
4-0	32	4	22
000	30	5	20
00	28	6	19
		7	18

B & S, Brown and Sharpe; *USP,* U.S. Pharmacopeia.

Flexon Steel Suture Material: Stainless Steel

Multistrand Flexon steel suture material is composed of 316L stainless steel conforming to ASTM Standard F138 grade 2 "stainless steel bar and wire for surgical implants." Steel sutures meet all requirements established by the USP (Table 4-1) and are characterized by the following (Fig. 4-16, *A* through *C*):

- Encapsulated in tissue
- Indicated for use in abdominal wound closure, intestinal anastomosis, hernia repair, sternal closure, and also for some orthopedic procedures (e.g., cerclage, tendon repair)
- Available in precut lengths, nonneedled or affixed to needles with permanent needle attachment techniques or ROTOGRIP
- Contraindicated in patients with known sensitivities or allergies to steel and its principal metallic components, chromium and nickel; additionally, the presence of steel may interfere with certain radiodiagnostics and its use is contraindicated where radiotransparency of suture is required
- Available in monofilament sizes 6-0 through 7 (metric sizes 0.7 to 9)

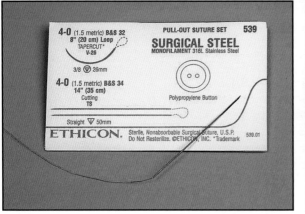
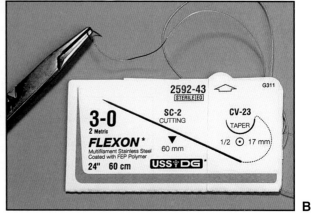

FIGURE **4-16** Stainless steel suture. (Courtesy Ethicon, 2004, Somerville, NJ. Reprinted from United States Surgical, a division of Tyco Healthcare Group, LP.) *Continued*

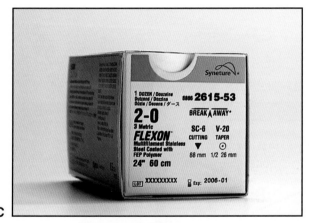

C

FIGURE **4-16** *Continued*

Multifilament Absorbable Suture Material
Synthetic
Vicryl/Polysorb Suture Material: Polyglactin 910

Vicryl/polysorb surgical suture material is synthetic, absorbable, and sterile. It is composed of a copolymer made from 90% glycolide and 10% L-lactide. Coated Vicryl is prepared by coating Vicryl suture material with a mixture composed of equal parts of copolymer of glycolide and lactide and calcium stearate. Polyglactin 910 copolymer and polyglactin 370 with calcium stearate have been found to be nonantigenic and nonpyrogenic. They elicit only a mild tissue reaction during absorption. Vicryl/polysorb suture material is available dyed or undyed (the latter of which is used for skin). It is characterized by the following (Fig. 4-17, *A* through *C*):

- 21-day wound support and an absorption rate of 56-70 days
- Indicated for use in gynecologic procedures, fascia closure, peritoneum, and skin
- Contraindicated in cardiovascular and neural tissue
- Available in precut lengths, ligating reels, and swaged-on and control-release needles
- Braided suture that is easy to handle with strong knot security
- Available in monofilament sizes 8-0 through 3 (metric sizes 0.4 to 6)

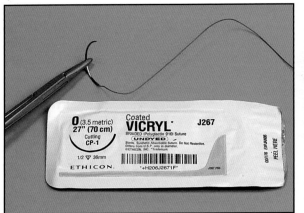
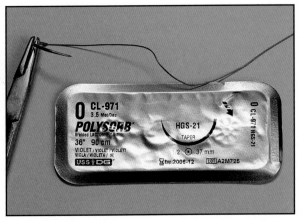

FIGURE **4-17** Vicryl/Polysorb suture. (Courtesy Ethicon, 2004, Somerville, NJ. Reprinted with permission of United States Surgical, a division of Tyco Healthcare Group, LP.)

Continued

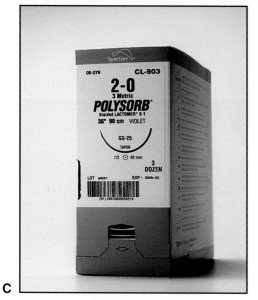

Coated Vicryl PLUS Suture Material: Polyglactin 910

Coated Vicryl PLUS surgical suture material is synthetic, absorbable, and sterile. It is composed of a copolymer made from 90% glycolide and 10% L-lactide. Coated Vicryl Plus Antibacterial suture material is coated with a mixture composed equally of a copolymer of glycolide and lactide and calcium stearate. The suture contains triclosan (Irgacare MP), a broad-spectrum antibacterial agent, and is characterized by the following (Fig. 4-18):

- 21-day wound support and an absorption rate of 56-70 days
- Indicated for use in gynecologic procedures, fascia closure, peritoneum, and skin
- Contraindicated in cardiovascular, ophthalmic, and neural tissue
- Available in precut lengths, ligating reels, swaged-on, and control-release needles
- Available dyed violet and undyed (natural)
- Braided suture that is easy to handle with strong knot security
- Available in monofilament sizes 5-0 through 0

C

FIGURE **4-17** *Continued*

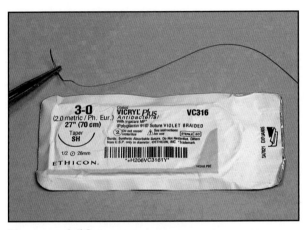

FIGURE **4-18** Vicryl plus suture. (Courtesy Ethicon, 2004, Somerville, NJ.)

Vicryl RAPIDE Suture Material: Polyglactin 910

Vicryl RAPIDE surgical suture material is synthetic, absorbable, and sterile. It is composed of a copolymer made from 90% glycolide and 10% L-lactide. Although this suture material is synthetic, it is designed to mimic the performance of plain gut suture. Characteristics follow (Fig. 4-19):

- 5-day wound support and an absorption rate of 42 days
- Indicated for use in superficial skin surfaces
- Contraindicated in cardiovascular, ophthalmic, and neural tissue
- Available in swaged-on needles
- Available undyed (natural)
- Braided suture that is easy to handle with strong knot security
- Available in monofilament sizes 5-0 through 1 (metric size 1 to 4)

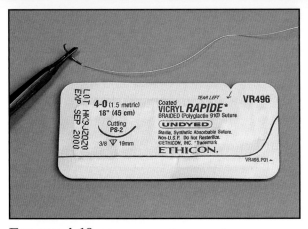

FIGURE **4-19** Vicryl RAPIDE suture. (Courtesy Ethicon, 2004, Somerville, NJ.)

Dexon II Suture Material: Polycaprolate

The synthetic, absorbable Dexon II suture material is composed of a copolymer of glycolic acid and coated with polycaprolate, a copolymer of glycolide and epsilon-caprolactone. It is characterized by the following (Fig. 4-20):

- 21-day wound support and an absorption rate of 60 to 90 days
- Indicated for use in general soft tissue approximation or ligation, or both, including ophthalmic procedures
- Contraindicated in cardiovascular and neural tissue
- Available in swaged-on needles
- Available undyed (beige), green dyed, or bicolor to enhance visibility in tissue
- Braided suture that is easy to handle with strong knot security

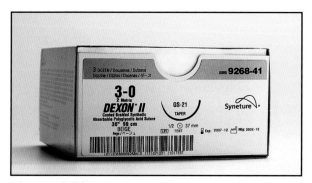

Figure 4-20 Dexon II suture. (Courtesy United States Surgical, a division of Tyco Healthcare Group, LP.)

Bondek Suture Material

The braided, synthetic, absorbable Bondek suture material is made of polyglycolic acid with a patented Polyglyd coating. It is characterized by the following:

- Absorption rate of 7 to 14 days
- Indicated for use in cosmetic and general closure
- Contraindicated in cardiovascular or neural tissue
- Polyglycolic acid breaks down evenly with predictability
- Braided suture that is easy to handle with strong knot security
- Available in precut lengths and swaged-on needles
- Bondek is available in sizes 2 through 8-0
- Suture is dyed green and violet and is available undyed in beige

Multifilament Nonabsorbable Suture Material

Natural

Cotton Suture Material

Cotton suture material, which is twisted, is the weakest of all nonabsorbable sutures. It is characterized by the following (Fig. 4-21):

- Gains tensile strength when wet
- Indicated for use in retracting vessels in cardiovascular and pediatric surgery
- Also indicated for tying off the umbilicus of newborns
- Suture is undyed
- Also called *umbilical tape*

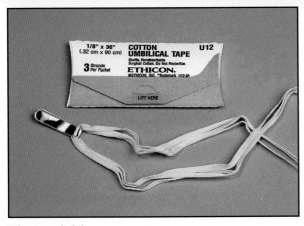

Figure **4-21** Cotton suture. (Courtesy Ethicon, 2004, Somerville, NJ.)

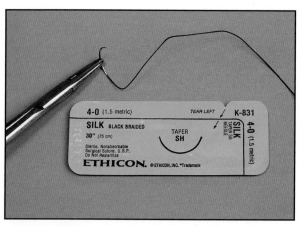

Figure **4-22** Silk suture. (Courtesy Ethicon, 2004, Somerville, NJ.)

Silk Suture Material

Perma-hand silk surgical suture material is nonabsorbable and sterile. It is composed of an organic protein called *fibroin* and is characterized by the following (Fig. 4-22):

- Indicated for use in gastrointestinal tissue and sometimes blood vessels or eye procedures
- Contraindicated in kidney, urinary bladder, gallbladder as it is a nucleus for stone formation
- Suture is available in virgin white or dyed black
- Suture is available in sizes 9-0 through 5 (metric sizes 0.3 to 7)
- Suture is supplied in swaged needles, ligating reels, and control release

SOFSILK Wax-Coated or Silicone-Treated Suture Material

SOFSILK surgical suture material is nonabsorbable, sterile, and nonmutagenic. It is composed of natural proteinaceous silk fibers called *fibroin*. The protein is derived from the domesticated silkworm, *Bombyx mori* species of the family Bombycidae. This suture material is characterized by the following (Fig. 4-23, *A* and *B*):

- Indicated for use in general soft tissue approximation or ligation, or both
- Contraindicated in kidneys, urinary bladder, and gallbladder nucleus (catalyst) or stone formation
- Indicated for use in cardiovascular, ophthalmic, and neurologic surgery and microsurgery
- Available in black with Logwood extract
- Available in sizes 9-0 through 5 (metric sizes 0.3 to 7)
- Supplied in swaged needles, ligating reels, and control release

Multifilament Nonabsorbable Suture
Synthetic
Nurolon Suture Material

Nurolon suture material is nonabsorbable, braided, and composed of aliphatic polymers Nylon 6 or Nylon 6.6. Nurolon sutures are dyed black to enhance visibility in tissue. They are also available undyed. Characteristics follow (Fig. 4-24):

- Indicated for use in general soft tissue approximation or ligation, or both
- Indicated for use in cardiovascular, ophthalmic, and neurologic surgery
- Nylon suture is dyed black
- Available in sizes 6-0 through 1 (metric sizes 0.7 to 4)

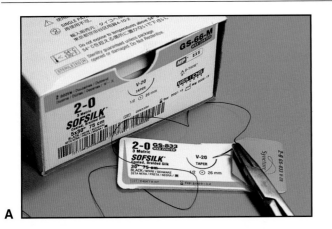

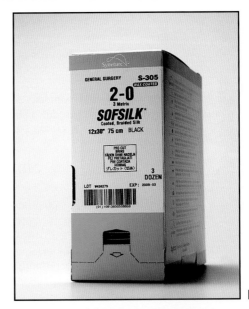

FIGURE **4-23** SOFSILK suture. (Courtesy United States Surgical, a division of Tyco Healthcare Group, LP.)

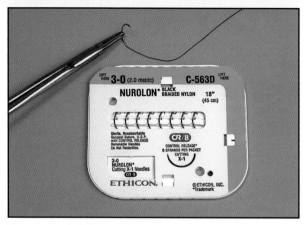

FIGURE **4-24** Nurolon suture. (Courtesy Ethicon, 2004, Somerville, NJ.)

- Available in sizes 4-0 through 1 (metric sizes 1.5 to 4) attached to control-release needles
- Supplied in swaged-on needles, ligating reels, and control-release needles

Surgilon Suture Material

Surgilon braided sutures are inert, nonabsorbable, and composed of Nylon 6 and Nylon 6.6. The braided sutures are coated uniformly with silicone to enhance handling characteristics, ease of passage through tissue, and reduction capillarity. They are characterized by the following (Fig. 4-25):

- Indicated for use in general soft tissue approximation or ligation, or both
- Also used in cardiovascular, ophthalmic, and neurologic surgery
- Available undyed (white) or dyed black
- Available in sizes 2 through 7-0 (metric sizes 5 to 0.5)
- Supplied in swaged-on needles, ligating reels, and control-release needles

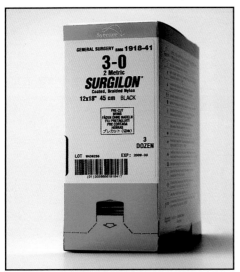

FIGURE **4-25** Surgilon suture. (Courtesy United States Surgical, a division of Tyco Healthcare Group, LP.)

Mersilene Suture Material

Mersilene is nonabsorbable, braided suture material composed of Poly (ethylene terephthalate). Mersilene sutures are braided for the best possible handling properties and may be dyed green for visibility. They are characterized by the following (Fig. 4-26):

- Indicated for use in general soft tissue approximation or ligation, or both
- Used in cardiovascular, ophthalmic, and neurologic surgery
- Available undyed (white) or monofilament dyed green
- Available in sizes 5 through 6-0 (metric sizes 7 to 0.7)
- Supplied in swaged-on needles and control-release needles

Ethibond Excel Suture Material

Ethibond is nonabsorbable, braided suture material composed of Poly (ethylene terephthalate). It is characterized by the following (Fig. 4-27):

- Indicated for use in general soft tissue approximation or ligation, or both
- Also used in cardiovascular, ophthalmic, and neurologic surgery to close incisions of the heart or to suture tendons in orthopedic

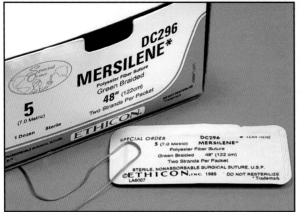

FIGURE 4-26 Mersilene. (Courtesy Ethicon, 2004, Somerville, NJ.)

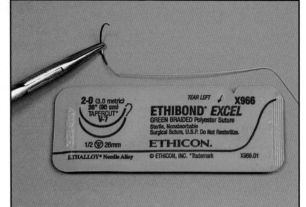

FIGURE 4-27 Ethibond suture. (Courtesy Ethicon, 2004, Somerville, NJ.)

- Available undyed (white) or dyed green
- Available in sizes 1 through 4-0 (metric sizes 1.5 to 4)
- Supplied in swaged-on needles and control-release needles

Ti-Cron Suture Material
Ti-Cron is braided, coated polyester suture material characterized by the following (Fig. 4-28, *A* and *B*):
- Indicated for use in general soft tissue approximation or ligation, or both
- Also used in cardiovascular, ophthalmic, and neurologic surgery to close incisions of the heart or to suture tendons in orthopedic surgery
- Available undyed (white) or dyed green
- Available in sizes 1 through 4-0 (metric sizes 1.5 to 4)
- Supplied in swaged-on needles and control-release needles

Tevdek/Polydek Suture Material
Both Tevdek and Polydek contain a PTFE coating that helps reduce "dead space," which renders the suture inert and reduces the possibility of wicking and tissue reactivity. These materials are characterized by the following:
- Tevdek was originally designed for heart valves implantation
- Polydek has a lighter PTFE treatment than Tevdek
- Cottony II is the uncoated version of this suture

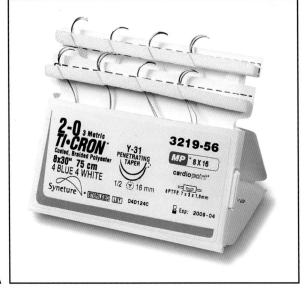

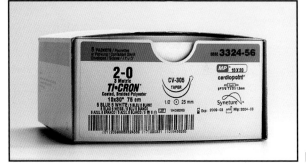

FIGURE **4-28** Ti-Cron suture. (Courtesy United States Surgical, a division of Tyco Healthcare Group, LP.)

- Available in sizes 9 through 10-0 (metric sizes 1.5 to 4)
- Dyed green and white for visibility
- Available braided and twisted

Surgidac Suture Material

Surgidac is braided, polyester, nonabsorbable suture material composed of Poly (ethylene terephthalate). It is characterized by the following:

- Indicated for use in general soft tissue approximation or ligation, or both
- Also used in cardiovascular, ophthalmic, and neurologic surgery
- Available undyed (white) or dyed green
- Available in sizes 5 through 8-0 (metric sizes 7 to 0.4)
- Supplied in swaged-on needles, ligating reels, and control-release needles

Suture Choice and Needle Use

Tissue Layers

Peritoneum

- Surgeon choice on closing peritoneum
- Possible suture: 0 PDS II or 0 or 2-0 Vicryl, 0 Chromic
- Needle: taper point

Gastrointestinal Tract

- Mucosa
  - Suture: coated synthetic absorbable such as Vicryl
  - Needle: taper point
- Serosa
  - Suture: synthetic absorbable suture
  - Needle: taper point
- Biliary tract
  - Suture: synthetic absorbable suture
  - Needle: taper point
- Oral cavity
  - Suture: synthetic absorbable suture
  - Needle: taper point
- Urinary tract
  - Suture: synthetic absorbable suture
  - Needle: taper point

Gynecology and Obstetrics

- Uterus
  - Suture: synthetic absorbable suture
  - Needle: taper point
- Uterine tube
  - Suture: coated synthetic absorbable suture
  - Needle: taper point
- Vaginal mucosa
  - Suture: coated synthetic absorbable suture
  - Needle: taper point

Vascular Surgery

- Grafts
  - Suture: braided coated polyester or polypropylene
  - Needle: taper point or taper cutting
- Arteriotomies
  - Suture: polypropylene
  - Needle: taper point or cutting

Orthopedic Surgery

- Synovial capsule
  - Suture: synthetic absorbable
  - Needle: taper point, taper cutting, or cutting
- Fibrous capsule
  - Suture: polypropylene
  - Needle: taper cutting
- Tendon
  - Suture: coated braided polyester or stainless steel
  - Needle: taper, taper cut, cutting, and trocar point

Suture Accessory Devices

CHAPTER 5

Retention Sutures

Retention or "stay" sutures are placed at a distance from the primary suture to relieve tension on the primary suture line. Heavy sutures are used in sizes that range from 0 to 5. Retention sutures can be placed in skin, subcutaneous tissue, and fascia. This includes rectus muscle and the peritoneum of an abdominal incision. Retention sutures are used often for patients in whom slow healing is expected due to malnutrition, obesity, carcinoma or infection; geriatric patients; patients receiving cortisone and even patients with respiratory problems. Retention sutures may be used as a preventive measure to prevent wound disruption on the primary suture line from distention, vomiting, or coughing postoperatively. Retention sutures are removed once the danger of intra-abdominal pressure is over.

Bridges

Bridges are plastic devices positioned on the skin to bridge the incision. The retention suture is brought up through the skin on both sides of the incision and through holes on each side of the bridge. Each side of the bridge has six holes spaced ¼ inch apart. The capstan on the bridge allows for adjustment of the tension as the incision heals. The suture is elevated from the skin, and pressure is evenly distributed over the incision (Fig. 5-1).

Bolster and Bumpers

Bolsters are surgical latex tubing. One end of the suture is threaded through the tubing before the suture is tied. The tubing covers all of the suture material that is on the skin surface. Compression bolsters are made from polyethylene foam held in place with malleable aluminum buttons to secure and distribute the tension of the suture (Fig. 5-2).

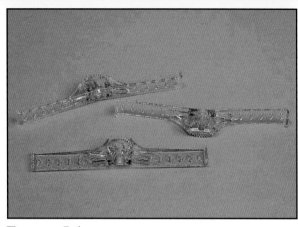

FIGURE **5-1** Suture bridge. (Courtesy Ethicon, 2004, Somerville, NJ.)

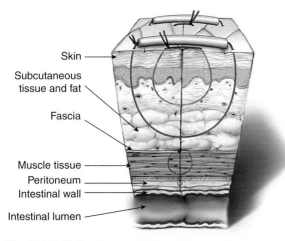

Skin

Subcutaneous
tissue and fat

Fascia

Muscle tissue
Peritoneum
Intestinal wall

Intestinal lumen

FIGURE 5-2 Suture bolster in abdominal wall. (From Sherris DA, Kern EB: *Essential surgical skills,* ed 2, Philadelphia, 2004, Saunders.)

Buttons and Beads

Buttons and beads are used to prevent suture from retracting or cutting into skin. Suture is pulled through the button hole and tied over the button. Beads may be positioned on the ends of pull-out subcuticular skin sutures (Fig. 5-3).

Traction Sutures

Traction sutures are used to retract tissue to the side or out of the way such as the tongue in a surgical procedure in the mouth. A nonabsorbable suture is placed through the tissue. Different materials may be used to retract or ligate vessels.

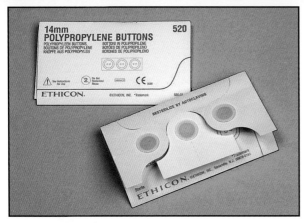

FIGURE **5-3** Suture buttons. (Courtesy Ethicon, 2004, Somerville, NJ.)

Umbilical Tape

Cotton umbilical tape may be used as a heavy tie or as a traction suture. It may be placed around a portion of bowel or a great vessel to retract it. Umbilical tape is a countable item and must be accounted for in its entirety (Fig. 5-4).

Vessel Loops

A length of flat silicone can be placed around a vessel, nerve, or other tubular structure for retraction. It can be made taut around a blood vessel for temporary vascular occlusion or for retraction of delicate structures. Vessel loops are colored for easy identification of structures. White or yellow loops are used on nerves or ducts, red loops for arteries, and blue loops for veins. Vessel loops are packaged in pairs and are countable items (Fig. 5-5).

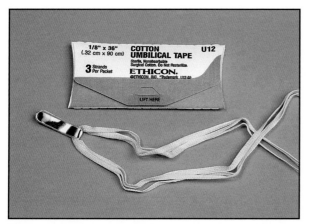

FIGURE 5-4 Umbilical tape. (Courtesy Ethicon, 2004, Somerville, NJ.)

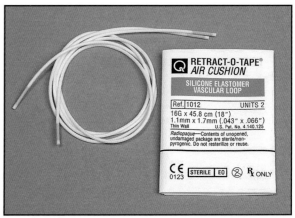

FIGURE 5-5 Vessel loops. (Courtesy Ethicon, 2004, Somerville, NJ.)

Adhesive Skin Closure Tapes

Adhesive skin closure tapes (Fig. 5-6) are adhesive-backed strips of nylon or polypropylene tape used to reinforce subcuticular skin closure or to approximate the wound edges of small incisions or lacerations. They have minimal tissue reactivity and a low rate of infection, although they slough off in the presence of tension or moisture.

Advantages of using skin adhesive tapes include no risk of needle-stick injuries, no tissue ischemia or necrosis, and rapid and simple closure. They have minimal tissue reactivity and have the lowest infection rate of any wound closure method. Adhesive skin tape cannot be used over oily or hair-bearing areas.

Topical Skin Adhesive

Topical skin adhesives can take the place of skin sutures where the skin is not pulled or stretched and where there is little or no body hair. Advantages of using skin adhesive include the following:
- Allows incisions to be closed three times faster than regular stitches
- Forms a protective barrier against infection-causing bacteria
- Is gentler to the skin than stitches
- Eliminates the need for bandages
- Provides the ability to shower

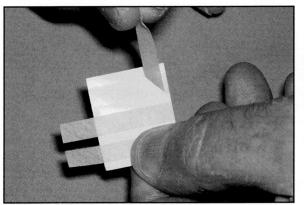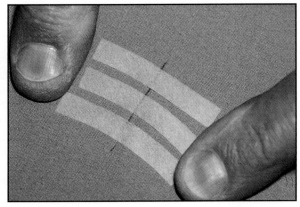

FIGURE **5-6** Adhesive skin closure tapes. (From Sherris DA, Kern EB: *Essential surgical skills,* ed 2, Philadelphia, 2004, Saunders.)

- Disappears as the wound heals
- Eliminates the need to remove stitches

Indermil (USS/DG, a division of United States Surgical) is one brand of topical skin adhesive. It is a sterile, liquid, topical tissue adhesive composed of n-butylo-2-cyanoacrylate monomer. Indermil is supplied in a 0.5-g, single-patient-use, plastic ampule. Each ampule is placed within a foil packet so that the exterior of the ampule is also sterile. Indermil can also be used with a Monoject BlunTip Safety I.V. Access Cannula (Kendall), which provides better visibility when applying it.

Indermil is applied to a dry wound with one layer of application to create an adhesive bond. Indermil also contains a microbial barrier. It seals in 30 seconds. Indermil remains liquid until exposed to water or water-containing substances/tissue, at which time it polymerizes and forms a film that bonds to the underlying surface (Fig. 5-7).

Dermabond (Ethicon) is a topical adhesive indicated for clean wounds that can be easily approximated. Dermabond works by using the moisture on the skin's surface to form a strong, flexible bond. It can be used in place of sutures, staples, or skin strips and in conjunction with deep dermal sutures.

Dermabond is made from 2-octyl cyanoacrylate, a liquid topical adhesive. The adhesive delivers a high viscosity that seals tissue in less than 3 minutes and provides strength of healed tissue at 7 days (Fig. 5-8).

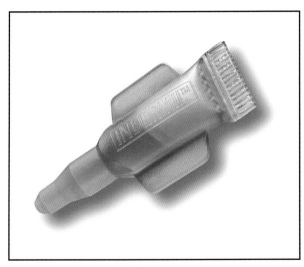

FIGURE **5-7** Indermil. (Courtesy United States Surgical, a division of Tyco Healthcare Group, LP.)

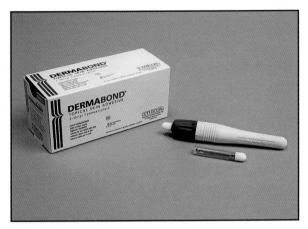

FIGURE **5-8** Dermabond. (Courtesy United States Surgical, a division of Tyco Healthcare Group, LP.)

Skin Staples

Staples can be used to approximate skin edges almost anywhere except the face.

Staples can be especially useful for closing scalp wounds, linear lacerations of the torso, and extremities. Skin staples are often used for closure of the abdomen and thorax. They are a rapid way to close skin with minimal harm or reaction to the patient. Staplers are for one-time use only and come in standard size (staples 35R) or wider size (staples 35W) (Fig. 5-9).

Tissue Repair Materials (Mesh)

Tissue deficiencies may require additional reinforcement or "bridging" in order to bring tissue together for proper closure. Mesh (Fig. 5-10) is also used to reinforce fascia defects. Synthetic mesh materials are used to fill congenital, traumatic, or acquired defects

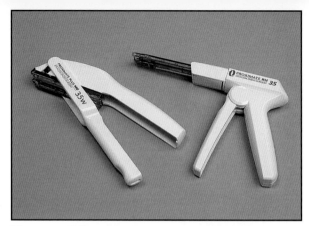

FIGURE **5-9** Skin staples. (Courtesy United States Surgical, a division of Tyco Healthcare Group, LP.)

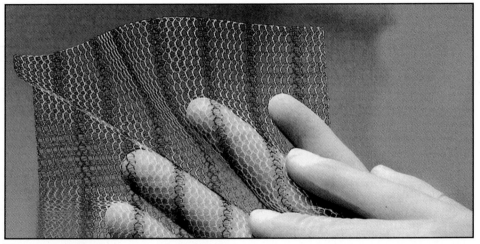

FIGURE 5-10 Mesh. (From Sherris DA, Kern EB: *Essential surgical skills,* ed 2, Philadelphia, 2004, Saunders.)

in fascia or a body wall and to reinforce fascia, as in a hernia repair. Synthetic meshes include the following:

- Polypropylene mesh: an inert material that can be used in the presence of infection. It has good elasticity and high tensile strength.
- Polyglactin 910 (Vicryl): absorbable mesh that offers temporary support during healing.
- Polytetrafluoroethylene (PTFE or Gore-Tex): a soft, flexible, nonabsorbable material. It should not be used when infection if present.
- Stainless steel mesh: rigid and difficult to work with. Although stainless steel mesh is the most inert material, it may cause discomfort in the patient if it fragments.
- Polyester fiber mesh (Mersilene): the least inert of the synthetic grafts. It should never be used in the presence of an infection, as the fiber construction may harbor bacteria.

Hemostasis

Hemostasis simply means the process of stopping bleeding. This can be achieved by clot formation or vessel spasm via mechanical means or topical application of hemostatic agents. When blood vessel injury occurs, the **endothelial** lining reacts by initiating **coagulation.** The arteries and arterioles, both of which comprise smooth muscle layers, react through **vasoconstriction** to reduce blood loss.

Topical Hemostasis

Topical hemostasis acts by chemical or mechanical means, or both, to produce hemostasis. The body ultimately absorbs the topical hemostatic agents.

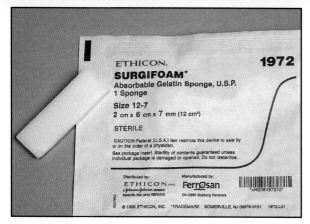

FIGURE **6-1** Sponge (Surgifoam). (Courtesy Ethicon, 2004, Somerville, NJ.)

Gelatin

Gelatin is available in either powder or compressed pad form (Gelfoam). As a pad, it is available in an assortment of sizes that can be cut as desired. As the gelatin swells, it absorbs blood to control oozing. It can absorb 45 times its own weight in blood. Gelatin is often soaked in thrombin or epinephrine solution. The gelatin adheres to platelets and enhances platelet formation (Figs. 6-1 and 6-2).

Oxidized Cellulose

Nu-Knit or Surgicel oxidized cellulose is available in the form of a pad or fabric. Blood clots quickly with cellulose, and the products form a gel that aids in hemostasis. The products can be wrapped around or held firmly against a bleeding site or laid dry on an oozing surface until hemostasis is obtained (Fig. 6-3).

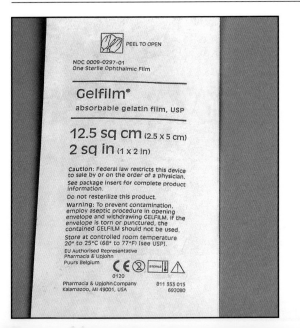

PEEL TO OPEN

NDC 0009-0297-01
One Sterile Ophthalmic Film

Gelfilm®

absorbable gelatin film, USP

12.5 sq cm (2.5 x 5 cm)
2 sq in (1 x 2 in)

Caution: Federal law restricts this device to sale by or on the order of a physician.
See package insert for complete product information.

Do not resterilize this product.

Warning: To prevent contamination, employ aseptic procedure in opening envelope and withdrawing GELFILM. If the envelope is torn or punctured, the contained GELFILM should not be used.

Store at controlled room temperature 20° to 25°C (68° to 77°F) [see USP].

EU Authorised Representative
Pharmacia & Upjohn
Puurs Belgium

CE 0120

Pharmacia & Upjohn Company
Kalamazoo, MI 49001, USA

811 353 015
692080

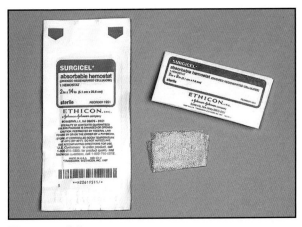

FIGURE 6-3 Surgicel. (Courtesy Ethicon, 2004, Somerville, NJ.)

Absorbable Collagen

Absorbable collagen (Collastat, Superstat, Helistat) or felt (Lyostypt) of bovine collagen origin are applied dry to oozing or bleeding sites. The collagen triggers the coagulation mechanism. The material dissolves as hemostasis happens. Any remaining collagen is absorbed in the wound. Collagen must be kept dry and should be applied with dry gloves or instruments. Absorbable collagen is contraindicated in the presence of infection or in areas where blood or other fluids have pooled (Fig. 6-4).

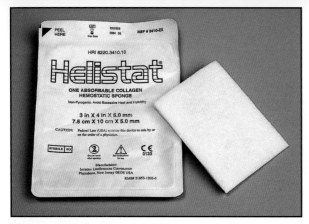

FIGURE **6-4** Helistat. (Courtesy Ethicon, 2004, Somerville, NJ.)

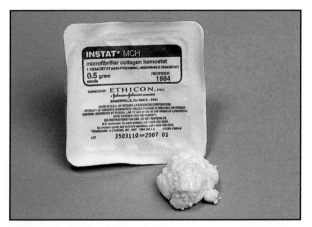

FIGURE **6-5** Microfibrillar collagen hemostat (Instat). (Courtesy Ethicon, 2004, Somerville, NJ.)

Microfibrillar Collagen

Microfibrillar collagen is available in compacted, nonwoven form or in loose fibrous form. Microfibrillar collagen (Avitene, Instat, Fig. 6-5) is a topical hemostatic agent. It is produced from a hydrochloric acid salt of purified bovine corium collagen and should be applied dry. The collagen traps platelets and induces the coagulation cascade producing the fibrin clot. Excess material should be removed from around the site. Microfibrillar collagen is supplied as spongelike sheets, pads, and felt (Avitene).

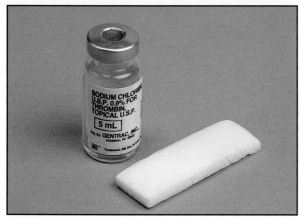

FIGURE **6-6** Thrombin.

Thrombin

Thrombin (topical thrombin U.S. Pharmacopeia) is derived from animal (bovine) blood. Thrombin accelerates clot formation by quickly converting fibrinogen into a fibrin clot within seconds. Thrombin is available as a powder and may be sprinkled on an oozing surface or put into isotonic saline and sprayed on areas of capillary bleeding. It is also saturated into a Gelfoam pad or collagen sponge. Thrombin should be mixed just before it is used because it will lose its potency after several hours. Thrombin should *never* be injected (Fig. 6-6).

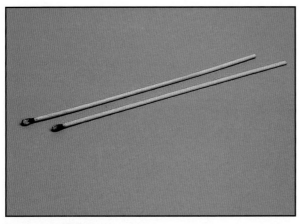

FIGURE **6-7** Silver nitrate.

Silver Nitrate

Silver nitrate is available as a solution or mixed with silver chloride and formed on applicator sticks that can be applied topically. Both an astringent and an antimicrobial, silver nitrate is often used in the treatment of burns (Fig. 6-7).

Epinephrine

Epinephrine, which may work on one or more adrenergic sites, promotes central nervous system and cardiac stimulation and bronchodilation. Epinephrine, also called *adrenalin,* is prepared synthetically to be used as a vasoconstrictor to prolong the action of local anesthetic agents to decrease bleeding. It may also counteract cardiovascular depressant effects of large doses of local anesthetic. Epinephrine is also used to treat allergic reaction, anaphylaxis, bronchospasm, or cardiac arrest.

Bone Wax

Bone wax is made from refined bee's wax and placed on the edge of bone as a mechanical barrier to seal oozing blood. It is often placed on a freer elevator and passed to the surgeon. Bone wax is used in thoracic surgery, as well as neurosurgery, orthopedic, and otorhinolaryngologic procedures (Fig. 6-8).

Pledgets

Pledgets are small squares of Teflon that can be used as a buttress over a bleeding suture line. Pledgets can be sewn over the hole in a vessel and can exert outside pressure over any of the small holes (Fig. 6-9).

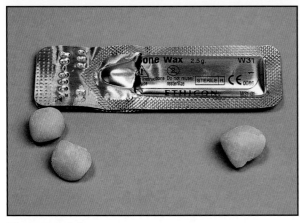

FIGURE **6-8** Bone wax. (Courtesy Ethicon, 2004, Somerville, NJ.)

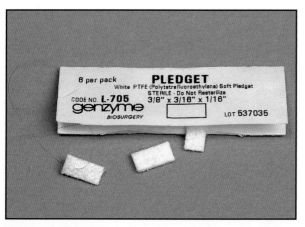

FIGURE **6-9** Pledgets.

Fibrin Glue

Fibrinogen and fibrin play a major role in wound healing and blood coagulation. As far back as 1909, fibrin powder was used to seal the wall of a blood vessel. In cerebral surgery, fibrin was used as early as 1915. Fibrinogen has been used to unite peripheral nerves. During the late 1970s fibrin glue was used effectively in sealing dural defects, splenic rupture, and visceral organ tears. In 1976 it was used in cardiac surgery. Fibrin glue has been found to be effective in bone repair, wound healing, nerve grafting, and for sealing mastoid and frontal cavities. More recently, fibrin glue has been used in virtually all surgical areas for hemostasis or tissue union.

Indications for fibrin glue follow:

- Controlling bleeding and approximating tissues that are difficult to approximate by suturing, such as liver, spleen, and lung

- Microsurgical anastomosis of blood vessels
- Reconstruction of middle ear
- Repair ocular implants
- Close superficial lacerations and fistula tracts
- May be used as a carrier for demineralized bone powder to promote osteoregeneration
- Repair dural tears

Fibrin Glue and Sealants

Fibrin glue and sealant components are fibrinogen, cryoprecipitated from human plasma; calcium chloride; and reconstituted thrombin of bovine origin. When applied topically to tissues, thrombin rapidly converts fibrinogen to fibrin to produce a clot (Fig. 6-10).

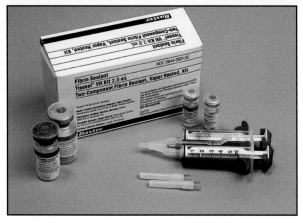

FIGURE **6-10** Fibrin glue. (Courtesy Ethicon, 2004, Somerville, NJ.)

Tisseel VH Fibrin Sealant

Tisseel VH fibrin sealant is characterized by the following:

- Is an adjunct to hemostasis for surgeries involving cardiopulmonary bypass and treatment of splenic injuries due to blunt or penetrating trauma to the abdomen where hemostasis by commonly used methods is ineffective
- Uses natural fibrin power
- Seals tissue with fibrinogen that converts to fibrin
- Creates netlike matrices to create stable watertight tissue seals
- Adheres to connective tissue
- Is effective in fully heparinized patients undergoing cardiopulmonary bypass
- *Must never be injected into tissues or vessels*

FloSeal Hemostatic Sealant

FloSeal hemostatic sealant is characterized by the following:

- Is indicated in surgical procedures (other than ophthalmic) as an adjunct to hemostasis when control of bleeding by conventional methods is ineffective or impractical
- Works on wet, actively bleeding tissue
- Requires only adequate circulating fibrinogen

- Does not require platelet activation
- Conforms to irregular surfaces
- Is bioresorbable/biocompatible
- Is of bovine origin
- *Must not be injected into blood vessels or allowed to enter blood vessels*

COSEAL Surgical Sealant

COSEAL surgical sealant is characterized by the following:
- Is a completely synthetic vascular sealing agent
- Is indicated for use in vascular reconstruction to achieve adjunctive hemostasis by mechanically sealing areas of leakage
- Seals almost immediately
- Should not be used in place of sutures, staples, or mechanical closure
- Swells up to four times its volume within 24 hours of application, and additional swelling may occur as the gel reabsorbs
- Has no known contraindications
- *Must not be injected into vessels*

Vessel Sealing Technology

The LigaSure system by Valleylab offers the surgeon a new option of ligating vessels and tissue bundles in general, gynecologic, urologic, and laparoscopic surgery. The hemostasis device works by fusing the collagen and elastin in vessels to seal the blood flow and allowing the vessel to be ligated.

The LigaSure generator incorporates Valleylab's patented Instant Response technology. This is a feedback controlled response system that diagnoses the tissue type in the jaws of the instrument and delivers the appropriate amount of energy to effectively seal the vessel or tissue bundle. When the seal cycle is complete, the generator tone sounds and output to the hand piece is automatically discontinued.

Several features make this a unique system for ligating vessels:
- It uses a combination of pressure and pulsed energy to create vessel fusion
- It uniformly fuses tissue bundles and vessels up to and including 7 mm in diameter without dissection or isolation
- It reduces thermal spread with less than 1 mm on isolated vessels
- It results in virtually no sticking or charring of tissue
- The generator uses a "plug and play" system that recognizes the type of PlasmaKinetic instrument that automatically sets the appropriate output for the instrument (Fig. 6-11, *A* through *F*)

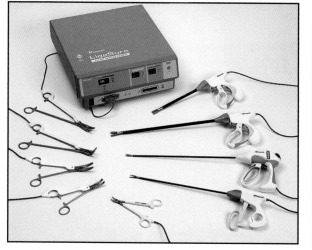
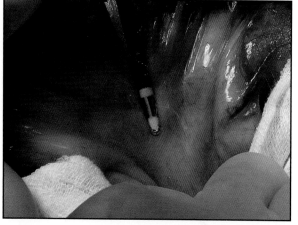

FIGURE **6-11** A through **F,** LigaSure system. (Courtesy Valleylab, a division of Tyco Healthcare Group, LP.)

Continued

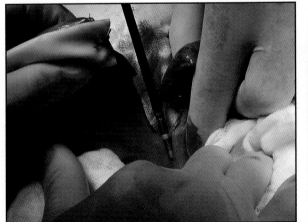
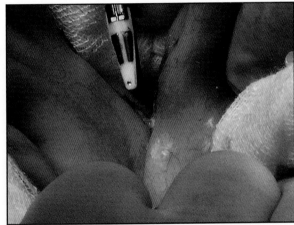

FIGURE **6-11** *Continued*

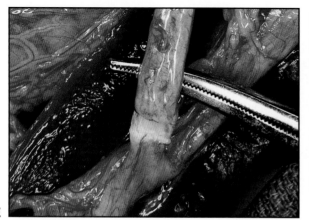

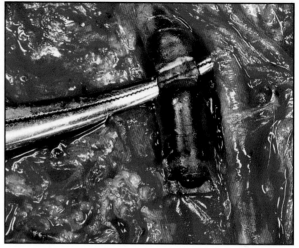

FIGURE **6-11** *Continued*

CHAPTER 7

Surgical Staples

History

The importance of leakproof anastomosis and hemostatic wound closure has been well documented. For centuries, using suture material was the only way to anastomose tissue. In 1826 Henroz of Belgium created a device with two rings that allowed the approximation of tissue from two bowel segments. In 1909 Hültl of Budapest redefined the principles of surgical stapling. Hültl and Fischer created an instrument that would be used to close the stomach during gastrectomies. In 1921 von Petz, a Hungarian surgeon, created a light and easy-to-use instrument that was easily adapted in the surgical field. Friedrich and Neuffer of Germany further improved upon this instrument. The main changes to the stapling device were simultaneous tissue compression and staple firing, along with the creation of cartridges that would allow the instrument to be used several times during the same operation. Nakayama of Japan further improved the stapler, yet staples were still not placed in a staggered fashion.

The next phase of development began at the end of World War II in Moscow. Due to the war, the decline in the number of surgeons led to thousands of deaths. Because hospitals and care centers were few and far between, there was a need for instruments for surgeons to use to perform surgical procedures quickly during emergencies. This was the reason for the creation of the Scientific Institute for Surgical Devices and Instruments.

In the 1950s the institute developed the following mechanical stapling devices, which were adopted throughout the Union of Soviet Socialist Republics:

- Linear staplers with reloadable cartridges using stainless steel staples
- Instruments to create side-by-side anastomoses between two bowel lumens
- Instruments to create end-to-end, end-to-side, or side-to-end circulator anastomoses

The third phase of development in stapling transpired when Mark Ravitch, an American surgeon, developed a new series of American instruments after a visit to Kiev. These instruments included reusable staplers with plastic preloaded staple cartridges that were sterilized and packaged for single use. The staplers were lighter and easier to use and could deliver different lengths of staple lines. All the instruments including the circular stapler delivered a double staggered row of staples, which was not available with the first generation of Russian instruments.

By the 1970s surgeons' awareness of the possibility of cross-contamination led to the development of single-patient-use staplers. Ethicon created the first skin stapler in 1976. In 1989 stainless steel staples and clips were replaced with titanium. Titanium is more biocompatible, allowing for less distortion of radiologic examinations (magnetic resonance imaging [MRI], plain films, and nuclear medicine).

Principles of Surgical Stapling

The basic requirements for an anastomosis are the following:
- Preservation of adequate tissue vascularization
- Creation of an adequate lumen
- Prevention of leakage and fistulas
- Evading of tissue tension
- Hemostasis

Advantages of Staplers

- Less tissue reaction
- Accelerated wound healing
- Efficiency
- Less anesthesia and operating room time

Types of Staplers
Linear Staplers

Linear staplers insert two straight or staggered, evenly spaced double rows of staples into tissue. Linear staplers allow the closure of organs at a line of transection. The tissue that is to be stapled is placed in the jaws of the stapler (Figs. 7-1 and 7-2).

Linear Cutters

Linear cutters have applications in gastrointestinal, gynecologic, thoracic, and pediatric surgery to transect, as well as resect, tissues. They are also used to create different types of anastomoses. Linear cutters should not be used on ischemic or necrotic tissue. Gastrointestinal anastomosis linear cutters can be reloaded seven times during a single procedure (Figs. 7-3 and 7-4).

Circular or Intraluminal Staplers

Circular or intraluminal staplers are used in gastrointestinal surgery to assist inverted end-to-end, end-to-side, side-to-end, and side-to-side anastomoses. Circular staplers offer a circular, double-staggered row of staples, while simultaneously creating a uniform stoma between the organs to be anastomosed. Circular staplers are not reloadable (Figs. 7-5 and 7-6).

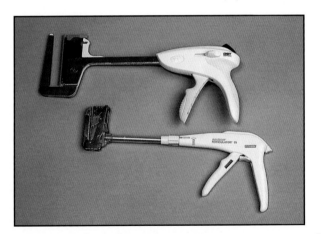

FIGURE **7-1** TA-30 and TA-90 (translinear anastomosis). (Courtesy United States Surgical, a division of Tyco Healthcare Group, LP.)

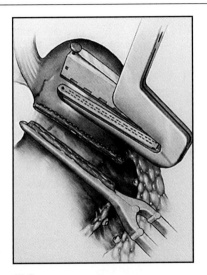

FIGURE **7-2** Closure of a gastric pouch using a TA linear stapler. (From Rothrock J: *Alexander's care of the patient in surgery,* ed 12, St Louis, 2002, Mosby.)

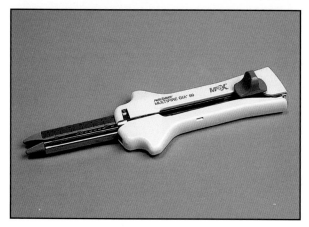

FIGURE **7-3** Gastrointestinal anastomosis instrument. (Courtesy United States Surgical, a division of Tyco Healthcare Group, LP.)

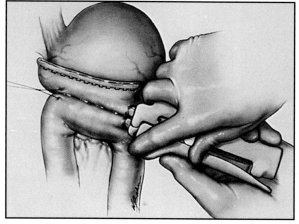

FIGURE **7-4** Use of GIA to staple and join stomach and jejunum. (From Rothrock J: *Alexander's care of the patient in surgery,* ed 12, St Louis, 2002, Mosby.)

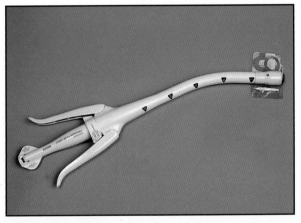

FIGURE **7-5** End-to-end anastomosis stapler. (Courtesy
United States Surgical, a division of Tyco Healthcare
Group, LP.)

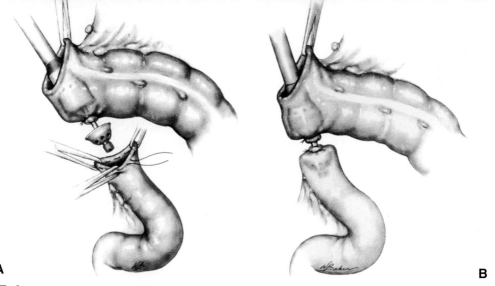

A

B

FIGURE **7-6** Hemicolectomy using the end-to-end anastomosis instrument to perform anastomosis. (Courtesy United States Surgical, a division of Tyco Healthcare Group, LP.)

Surgical Staples

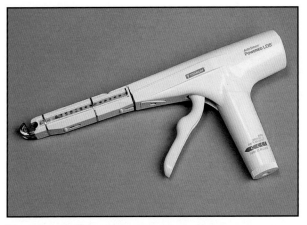

FIGURE **7-7** Ligating and dividing stapler. (Courtesy United States Surgical, a division of Tyco Healthcare Group, LP.)

Ligating and Dividing Stapler

A ligating and dividing stapler (LDS) issues a double row of two staples and ligates the tissues, which are then divided simultaneously between the staple lines. The LDS stapler is often used for separating tissue planes such as the omentum (Figs. 7-7 and 7-8).

Purse-String Suture Clamp

A purse-string suture clamp assists prompt placement of a purse-string suture (Figs. 7-9 and 7-10).

Skin Staplers

Skin staplers are used to approximate skin edges by firing a single staple with each squeeze of the trigger. Edges of both cuticular and subcuticular layers are aligned with the edges slightly raised. Skin staplers are supplied preloaded with different quantities of staples in varying widths.

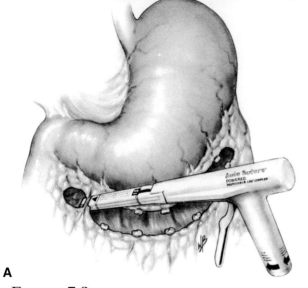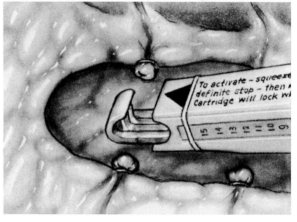

FIGURE **7-8** Use of a ligating and dividing stapler. (Courtesy United States Surgical, a division of Tyco Healthcare Group, LP.)

Surgical Staples

208

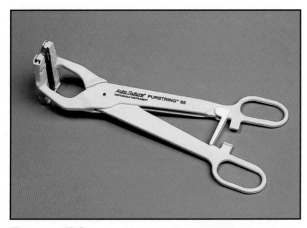

FIGURE **7-9** Purse-string stapler. (Courtesy United States Surgical, a division of Tyco Healthcare Group, LP.)

Skin staples are removed 5 to 7 days postoperatively (Fig. 7-11).

Multiple Clip Appliers

Multiple clip appliers are designed to provide quick, efficient ligation by an automatic reloadable applier with a ratchet that prevents clips from being displaced from the jaws accidentally (Fig 7-12).

Hem-O-Lok Ligating Clips

In 1999 Weck Closure Systems offered the Hem-o-lok polymer ligating clip. This clip is designed to eliminate clip dropout from the appliers, improve security of the clip on vessels, provide tactile closure feedback to surgeons, and eliminate imaging interference with MRI and computed tomography scans. The Hem-o-lok successfully ligates through a variety of tissues that

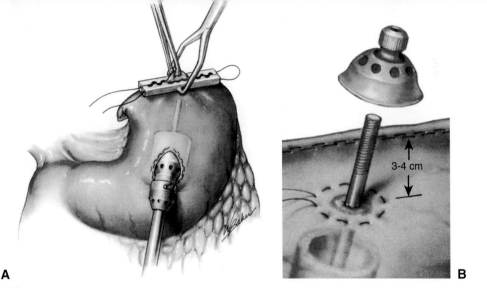

FIGURE **7-10** Placement of a purse-string suture to accommodate the anvil of the circular end-to-end anastomosis stapler. (Courtesy United States Surgical, a division of Tyco Healthcare Group, LP.)

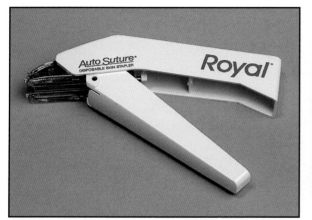

FIGURE **7-11** Skin stapler. (Courtesy United States Surgical, a division of Tyco Healthcare Group, LP.)

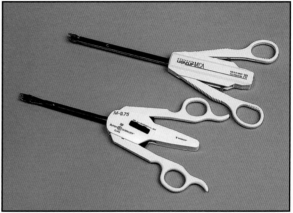

FIGURE **7-12** Clip appliers. (Courtesy United States Surgical, a division of Tyco Healthcare Group, LP.)

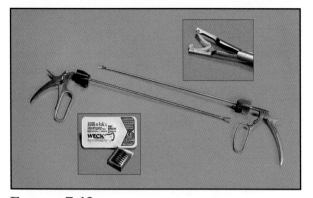

FIGURE **7-13** Hem-o-lok clip appliers. (Courtesy United States Surgical, a division of Tyco Healthcare Group, LP.)

surround blood vessels. The Hem-o-lok can also be used in minimally invasive surgery (Fig. 7-13).

Endoscopic Staplers

Endoscopic staplers have been developed for the various endoscopic procedures that are replacing traditional open surgeries. Ligating, dividing, and linear staplers exist (Figs. 7-14 and 7-15).

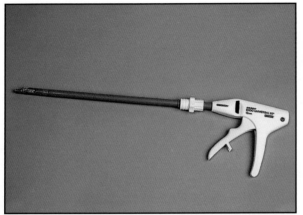

FIGURE **7-14** Endo gastrointestinal anastomosis used for laparoscopic procedures. (Courtesy United States Surgical, a division of Tyco Healthcare Group, LP.)

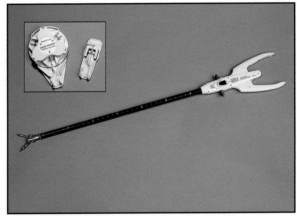

FIGURE **7-15** Endo stitch used for suturing laparoscopically.

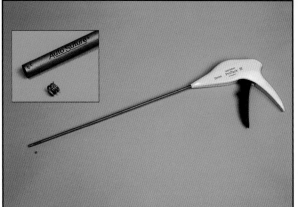

FIGURE **7-16** ProTack™ stapler used in laparascopic procedures to secure mesh.

Appendix A

Needle Conversion Chart

Ethicon	Syneture	Ethicon	Syneture
BB	CV-15	OS-4	HOS-10
BV	CV	OS-6	HOS-11
BV-1	CV-1	P-1	P-10
BV-75-4	MV-70-4	P-2	P-21
BV-100-4	MV-100-4	P-3	P-13
BV-130-5	MV-135-5	PC-1	PC-13
BV-175-6	MV-175-8	PC-3	PC-11
C-1	CV-11	PS-1	P-14
CC	KV-1	PS-2	P-12
CC-1	KV-11	PS-4	P-24
CCS	SCC	PS-5	P-22
CP	GS-12	RB-1	CV-23
CP-1	GS-11	RB-2	CV-22

Ethicon	Syneture	Ethicon	Syneture
CS-160-6	SE-160-6	S-2	SS-2
CT	GS-24	S-14	SS-14
CT-1	GS-21, HGS-21	S-29	SS-29
CT-2	GS-22	SH	V-20, GS-22
CTX	GS-25	SH-1	CV-25
FN-2	GS-23	TF	CVF-21
FS	C-15	TG-140-8	SE-140-8
FS-1	C-14	TP-1	GS-26
FS-2	C-13	UR-5	GU-45
FSL	C-16	UR-6	GU-46
G-1	HE-1	V-4	KV-15
G-3	HE-3	V-5	KV-5
G-6	HE-6	V-7	KV-7
KS	SC-2	V-34	KV-34
MH	V-26	V-37	KV-37
MO-4, CT-1	HGS-21	V-40	KV-40
MO-6	HGS-22	X-1	C-23

Courtesy of Ethicon, Inc., 2004, Somerville, NJ; reprinted with permission of United States Surgical, a division of Tyco Healthcare Group, LP.

Appendix B

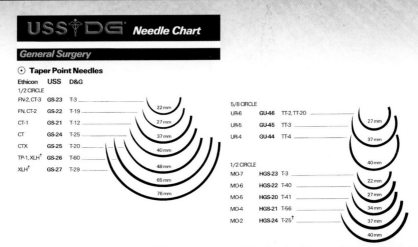

USS DG Needle Chart

General Surgery

⊙ Taper Point Needles

1/2 CIRCLE

Ethicon	USS	D&G	
FN-2, CT-3	GS-23	T-3	22 mm
FN, CT-2	GS-22	T-19	27 mm
CT-1	GS-21	T-12	37 mm
CT	GS-24	T-25	40 mm
CTX	GS-25	T-20	48 mm
TP-1, XLH†	GS-26	T-60	65 mm
XLH†	GS-27	T-29	76 mm

5/8 CIRCLE

UR-6	GU-46	TT-2, TT-20	27 mm
UR-5	GU-45	TT-3	37 mm
UR-4	GU-44	TT-4	40 mm

1/2 CIRCLE

MO-7	HGS-23	T-3	22 mm
MO-6	HGS-22	T-40	27 mm
MO-5	HGS-20	T-41	34 mm
MO-4	HGS-21	T-56	37 mm
MO-2	HGS-24	T-25†	40 mm

Blunt Point Needles

1/2 CIRCLE

CTB-1	**BGS-21**	MT-12	37 mm
—	**BGS-24**	MT-25	40 mm
CTX-B	**BGS-25**	MT-20	48 mm
BP-1	**BGS-29**	MT-60†	63 mm
—	**BGS-27**	BT-60	64 mm
BP	**BGS-28**	—	85 mm

3/8 CIRCLE

—	—	NE-9	64 mm

⊙ Straight Taper Point Needles

—	—	TS-4	44 mm
ST	**ST-1**	—	51 mm
ST-1	**ST**	TS-9	60 mm

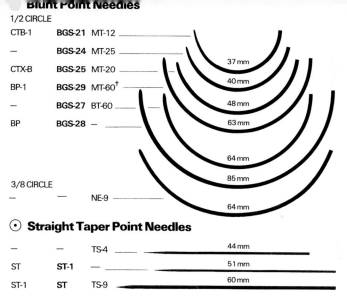

Cardiovascular

⊙ Taper Point Needles

Cardiovascular, Gastrointestinal, Pediatric

Ethicon	USS	D&G	
3/8 CIRCLE			
BV-1	CV-1, CVF-1	TE-10[†], TE-11[†]	9 mm
BV	CV, CVF	TE-9	11 mm
C-1	CV-11, CVF-11	TE-1[†]	13 mm
BB	CV-15	TE-7[†]	17 mm
BB-1	CV-13	—	22 mm
TE	CV-17	TE-3[†]	32 mm
—	CV-19	—	50 mm

			1/2 CIRCLE
RB-3[†]	CV-20	T-37, CV-337	10 mm
TF	CVF-21	T-30[†]	12 mm
RB-2	CV-22, CVF-22	T-30	13 mm
RB-1	CV-23, CVF-23	T-31, CV-331[†]	17 mm
SH-2	CV-24	T-16	20 mm
SH-1	CV-25	—	22 mm
SH	V-20, VF-20	T-5, CV-305[†]	26 mm
—	V-30	T-15	30 mm
MH	V-26	T-10	37 mm

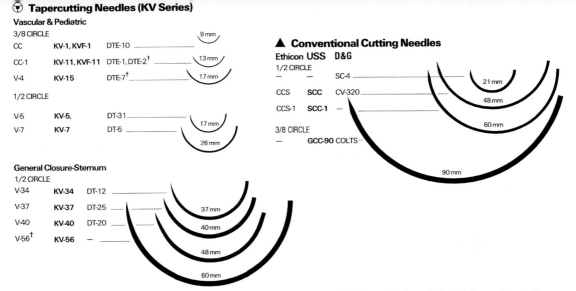

⊙ Tapercutting Needles (KV Series)

Vascular & Pediatric

3/8 CIRCLE

CC	**KV-1, KVF-1**	DTE-10	9 mm
CC-1	**KV-11, KVF-11**	DTE-1, DTE-2[†]	13 mm
V-4	**KV-15**	DTE-7[†]	17 mm

1/2 CIRCLE

V-5	**KV-5,**	DT-31	17 mm
V-7	**KV-7**	DT-5	26 mm

General Closure-Sternum

1/2 CIRCLE

V-34	**KV-34**	DT-12	37 mm
V-37	**KV-37**	DT-25	40 mm
V-40	**KV-40**	DT-20	48 mm
V-56[†]	**KV-56**	—	60 mm

▲ Conventional Cutting Needles

Ethicon	USS	D&G	
1/2 CIRCLE			
—	—	SC-4	21 mm
CCS	**SCC**	CV-320	48 mm
CCS-1	**SCC-1**	—	60 mm
3/8 CIRCLE			
—	**GCC-90**	COLTS—	90 mm

Plastic/Cosmetic

▼ Premium Reverse Cutting Needles

3/8 CIRCLE

P-6	**P-16**	PRE-20	7 mm
P-1	**P-10**	PRE-1, SBE-1	11 mm
P-3	**P-13**	PRE-2, SBE-2, PRE-302	13 mm
PS-3	**P-11**	PRE-3, SBE-3	16 mm
PS-2	**P-12**	PRE-4, SBE-4, PRE-304	19 mm
PS-1	**P-14**	PRE-6, SBE-6	24 mm

1/2 CIRCLE

P-2	**P-21**	PR-1, C-1	9 mm
PS-5	**P-22**	PR-2	13 mm
PS-4	**P-24**	PR-4†	16 mm

▲ Premium Conventional Cutting Needles

3/8 CIRCLE

PC-1†	**PC-13**	PE-1†	11 mm
PC-3	**PC-11**	PE-3	16 mm
PC-5	**PC-12**	PE-5	19 mm

Orthopedic

▼ Reverse Cutting Needles
General Closure

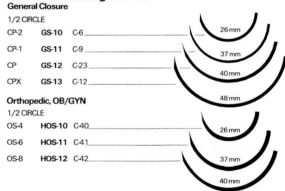

1/2 CIRCLE

CP-2	**GS-10**	C-6	26 mm
CP-1	**GS-11**	C-9	37 mm
CP	**GS-12**	C-23	40 mm
CPX	**GS-13**	C-12	48 mm

Orthopedic, OB/GYN
1/2 CIRCLE

OS-4	**HOS-10**	C-40	26 mm
OS-6	**HOS-11**	C-41	37 mm
OS-8	**HOS-12**	C-42	40 mm

▼ Reverse Cutting Needles

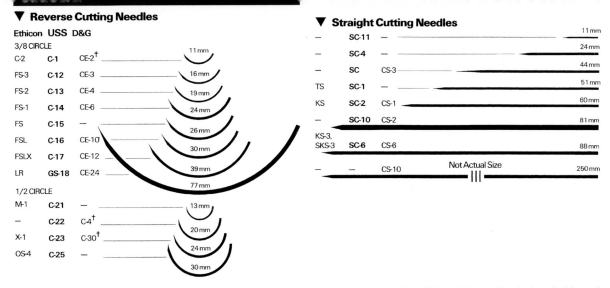

Ethicon USS D&G

3/8 CIRCLE

Ethicon	USS	D&G
C-2	C-1	CE-2†	11 mm
FS-3	C-12	CE-3	16 mm
FS-2	C-13	CE-4	19 mm
FS-1	C-14	CE-6	24 mm
FS	C-15	—	26 mm
FSL	C-16	CE-10	30 mm
FSLX	C-17	CE-12	
LR	GS-18	CE-24	39 mm
			77 mm

1/2 CIRCLE

Ethicon	USS	D&G
M-1	C-21	—	13 mm
—	C-22	C-4†	20 mm
X-1	C-23	C-30†	24 mm
OS-4	C-25	—	30 mm

▼ Straight Cutting Needles

—	SC-11	—	11 mm
—	SC-4	—	24 mm
—	SC	CS-3	44 mm
TS	SC-1	—	51 mm
KS	SC-2	CS-1	60 mm
—	SC-10	CS-2	81 mm
KS-3, SKS-3	SC-6	CS-6	88 mm
—	—	CS-10	Not Actual Size 250 mm

Appendix B

Microsurgery

⊙ Taper Point Needles

3/8 CIRCLE

BV-50-3/2[†]	MV-50-3	TE-50	4 mm
BV-75-3[†]	MV-70-3	TE-70	4 mm
BV-100-3	MV-100-3	TE-143	4 mm
BV-130-3	MV-135-3	TE-143	4 mm
BV-75-4	MV-70-4	TE-100	5 mm
BV-100-4	MV-100-4	TE-100	5 mm
BV-130-4/5[†]	MV-135-4	CV-345, TE-100	5 mm
BV-130-5	MV-135-5	CV-345, TE-145	6 mm
BV-175-6	MV-175-8	CV-351	8 mm
BV-175-6	MVF-175-8	CV-351	8 mm
BV-175-8	MV-175-9	TE-11, TE-10	10 mm

⊛ Tapercutting Needles

Ethicon	USS	D&G	
3/8 CIRCLE			
—	MVK-70-3	CTE-103	4 mm
V-100-3 V-130-3[†]	MVK-100-4	CTE-100	5 mm

Ophthalmic

● Premium Point Spatula Needles

1/4 CIRCLE

CS/TG-100-8	SE-100-8	LO-90-8	6 mm
3/8 CIRCLE			
CS/TG-140-6	SE-140-6	LE-140-6 (LE-1)	6 mm
CS/TG-140-8	SE-140-8	LE-140-8 (LE-2)	6 mm
1/2 CIRCLE			
CS/TG-160-4	SE-160-4	LA-160-4 (LA-100)	6 mm
CS/TG-160-6 TGW-160-6	SE-160-6	LA-160-6 (LA-1)	6 mm
CS/TG-160-8	SE-160-8	LA-160-8 (LA-2)	6 mm
CS/TG-175-8	SE-175-8	L-175-8 (L-2)	7 mm
COMPOUND CURVE			
CS-C-6[†]	SE-CC-6	LB-90/50-6	5 mm

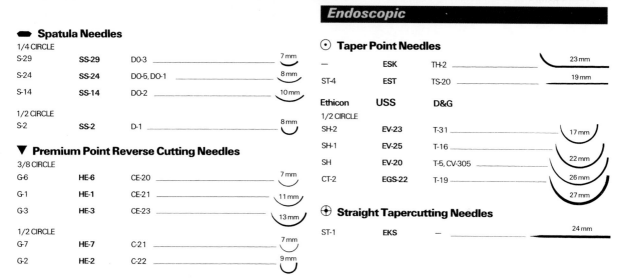

🖝 Spatula Needles

1/4 CIRCLE

S-29	**SS-29**	DO-3	7 mm
S-24	**SS-24**	DO-5, DO-1	8 mm
S-14	**SS-14**	DO-2	10 mm

1/2 CIRCLE

S-2	**SS-2**	D-1	8 mm

▼ Premium Point Reverse Cutting Needles

3/8 CIRCLE

G-6	**HE-6**	CE-20	7 mm
G-1	**HE-1**	CE-21	11 mm
G-3	**HE-3**	CE-23	13 mm

1/2 CIRCLE

G-7	**HE-7**	C-21	7 mm
G-2	**HE-2**	C-22	9 mm

Endoscopic

⊙ Taper Point Needles

—	**ESK**	TH-2	23 mm
ST-4	**EST**	TS-20	19 mm

Ethicon	USS	D&G	
1/2 CIRCLE			
SH-2	**EV-23**	T-31	17 mm
SH-1	**EV-25**	T-16	22 mm
SH	**EV-20**	T-5, CV-305	26 mm
CT-2	**EGS-22**	T-19	27 mm

⊕ Straight Tapercutting Needles

ST-1	**EKS**	—	24 mm

USS·DG· Product	Material	Ethicon
POLYSORB*	Coated, Braided Synthetic Absorbable	Vicryl (Coated)
DEXON* II DEXON* S	Coated and Uncoated Braided, Synthetic Absorbable	Vicryl (Coated)
BIOSYN*	Monofilament, Synthetic Absorbable	Monocryl
MAXON*	Monofilament, Synthetic Absorbable	PDS II
MILD & CHROMIC GUT	Natural Absorbable Gut	Surgical Gut
PLAIN GUT	Natural Absorbable Gut	Surgical Gut
SURGIPRO* SURGILENE*	Nonabsorbable, Monofilament Polypropylene	Prolene
NOVAFIL*	Nonabsorbable, Monofilament Polybutester	Prolene
VASCUFIL*	Nonabsorbable Monofilament Polybutester with Polytribolate Absorbable Coating	Pronova
SURGIDAC* Ti-CRON*	Nonabsorbable Coated Braided Polyester	Mersilene (Uncoated) Ethibond (Coated)
MONOSOF* DERMALON*	Nonabsorbable Monofilament Nylon	Ethilon
BRALON* SURGILON*	Nonabsorbable Coated Braided Nylon	Nurolon
SOFSILK* SILK	Nonabsorbable Coated Braided Silk	*Permahand* Silk (Coated)
STEEL	Nonabsorbable 316L Stainless Steel	Surgical Stainless Steel
FLEXON*	Temporary Cardiac Pacing Wire	Surgical Stainless Steel

Appendix C

Syneture Suture Products

Brand Name	Construction	Competitor
POLYSORB	Coated Braided Synthetic Absorbable	Vicryl (Coated)
BIOSYN	Monofilament Synthetic Absorbable	Monocryl
MAXON	Monofilament Synthetic Absorbable	PDSII
MILD & CHROMIC GUT	Natural Absorbable Gut	Chromic Gut
PLAIN GUT	Natural Absorbable Gut	Plain Gut
SURGIPRO	Nonabsorbable Monofilament Polypropylene	Prolene
TICRON	Nonabsorbable Coated Braided Polyester	Ethibond/Mersilene
MONOSOF	Nonabsorbable Monofilament Nylon	Ethilon
DERMALON		
SURGILON	Nonabsorbable Coated Braided Nylon	Nurolon
SOFSILK	Nonabsorbable Coated Braided Silk	Silk
STEEL	Nonabsorbable 316L Stainless Steel	Surgical Stainless Steel
FLEXON	Temporary Cardiac Pacing Wire	Pacing Wire

Syneture Suture Products *Continued*

Brand Name	Construction	Competitor
Alternative Suture Products		
DEXON II	Coated Braided Absorbable Synthetic	Vicryl (Coated)
DEXON S	Uncoated Braided Absorbable Synthetic	
CAPROSYN	Monofilament Synthetic Absorbable	Monocryl/gut
NOVAFIL	Nonabsorbable Monofilament Polybutester	Prolene/Ethilon
VASCUFIL	Nonabsorbable Monofilament Polybutester with Polytribolate Absorbable Coating	Prolene

Courtesy of Ethicon, Inc., 2004, Somerville, NJ; reprinted with permission of United States Surgical, a division of Tyco Healthcare Group, LP.

Syneture Absorbable Sutures

Indications	Brand Name	Construction	Duration	Length
Short-Term Wound Support	CAPROSYN	Monofilament	10 days	<56
Medium-Term Wound Support	POLYSORB	Braided, Coated	3 weeks	56-70
Medium-Term Wound Support	DEXON II	Braided, Coated	3 weeks	60-90
Medium-Term Wound Support	DEXON S	Braided, Uncoated	3 weeks	60-90
Medium-Term Wound Support	BIOSYN	Monofilament	3 weeks	90-110
Long-Term Wound Support	MAXON	Monofilament	6 weeks	180

Courtesy of Ethicon, Inc., 2004, Somerville, NJ; reprinted with permission of United States Surgical, a division of Tyco Healthcare Group, LP.

Syneture Non-absorbable Sutures

Type	Brand Name	Construction	Clinical Specialty Indications
Nylon	DERMALON	Monofilament	Cardiovascular, Ophthalmic and Neurological
Nylon	MONOSOF	Monofilament	Cardiovascular, Ophthalmic and Neurological
Nylon	SURGILON	Braided, Coated	Cardiovascular, Ophthalmic and Neural Tissue

Syneture Non-absorbable Sutures *Continued*

Type	Brand Name	Construction	Clinical Specialty Indications
Polyester	SURGIDAC	Braided, Coated	Cardiovascular, Ophthalmic and Neurological
Polyester	TI•CRON	Braided, Coated	Cardiovascular, Ophthalmic and Neural Tissue
Polypropylene	SURGIPRO	Monofilament	Cardiovascular, Ophthalmic and Neurological
Polypropylene	SURGIPRO II	Monofilament	Cardiovascular, Ophthalmic and Neurological
Polybutester	NOVAFIL	Monofilament	Cardiovascular and Ophthalmic
Polybutester	VASCUFIL	Monofilament, Coated	Cardiovascular and Ophthalmic
Silk	SOFSILK	Silk, Coated	Cardiovascular, Ophthalmic and Neurological
Steel	FLEXON	Multistrand	Cardiovascular
Steel	STEEL	Monofilament	Cardiovascular, General Surgery and Orthopedic

Courtesy of Ethicon, Inc., 2004, Somerville, NJ; reprinted with permission of United States Surgical, a division of Tyco Healthcare Group, LP.

Appendix D

Staple Size before Firing	Lengths and Color	Staple Size after Firing	PROBABLE USE: Tissue which can compress between:
2.0 mm	30 mm, 45 mm **GRAY***	0.75 mm	0.75 and 1.00 mm: Mesenteric vessels
2.5 mm	30 mm, 45 mm, 60 mm **WHITE**	1.00 mm	1.00 and 1.50 mm: Vascular tissue, small bowel and appendix
3.5 mm	30 mm, 45 mm, 60 mm **BLUE**	1.50 mm	1.50 and 2.00 mm: Colon, gastric tissue and lung
4.8 mm	45 mm, 60 mm **GREEN** -Straight Only-	2.00 mm	2.00 and 2.50 mm: Thick tissue, colon, lung, gastric tissue

ENDO GIA UNIVERSAL STAPLER TIPS:

The yellow shipping wedge must never be taken off until after the reload has been loaded onto the stapler!
The jaws of the reload must be open to unload.
To open jaws, pull the black return nobs back to proximal end of stapler.
Once loaded, squeeze handle to close, and pull return knobs back to open again.
If you can do this, then the stapler has been loaded correctly.
*Gray 2.0mm reloads only available with ENDO GIA/GIA Universal.

Cartridge lengths 30mm
40mm
60mm

Squeezes required to fully fire cartridge:

30mm = 2 full squeezes
45mm = 3 full squeezes
60mm = 4 full squeezes

Handle can be reloaded and fired 25 times.

Courtesy of Ethicon, Inc., 2004, Somerville, NJ; reprinted with permission of United States Surgical, a division of Tyco Healthcare Group, LP.

Glossary

Adhesion – A band of scar tissue that joins two anatomic surfaces that are not normally attached.

Adipose – Adipose tissue is composed of fat cells arranged in lobules.

Arrector pili muscle – The muscle that raises hair on the skin.

Atraumatic – Causing little or no trauma.

Breaking strength – The load required to break a wound regardless of its dimension.

Burst strength – The amount of pressure needed to rupture a viscus, or large interior organ.

Ceruminous – Modified sweat glands that produce a waxy substance known as cerumen. Also known as earwax.

Coagulation – The conversion of blood from a free flowing liquid to a semisolid gel.

Collagen – A protein consisting of bundles of tiny reticular fibrils, which combine to form the white glistening inelastic fibers of the tendons, the ligaments, and the fascia.

Continuous – Without interruption.

Cutaneous – Pertaining to the skin.

Cyanosis – Bluish discoloration of the skin and mucous membranes caused by an excess of deoxygenated hemoglobin in the blood or a structural defect in the hemoglobin molecule, such as in methemoglobin.

Dead space – A cavity that remains after the incomplete closure of a surgical or traumatic wound, leaving an area in which blood can collect and delay healing.

Debridement – removal of damaged tissue and cellular or other debris from a wound to promote healing and to prevent infection.

Ductility – The property of tissue that has a large elastic range and tends to deform before failing from stress.

Decubitus ulcers – An inflammation, sore, or ulcer in the skin over a bony prominence. It results from ischemic hypoxia of the tissues because of prolonged pressure on the part.

Dehiscence – partial or total splitting open or separation of the layers of a wound.

Edema – abnormal accumulation of fluid in interstitial spaces of tissues.

Efficacy – The maximum ability of a drug or treatment to produce a result, regardless of the dosage.

Electrocautery – The application of a needle or snare heated by electric current for the destruction of tissue.

Encapsulated – Enclosed in fibrous or membranous sheaths.

Endothelial – Pertaining to or resembling endothelium.

Evert – Turning outward of tissue.

Extracorpeal – Something that is outside the body.

Extravasation – passage of blood, serum, lymph into tissues.

Exudate – Fluid, cells, or other substances that have been discharged from vessels or tissues. It contains white blood cells, lymphocytes, and growth factors that stimulate healing.

Eviseration – Protrusion of viscera through an abdominal incision.

Fibroblasts – A flat, elongated undifferentiated cell in the connective tissue that gives rise to various precursor cells.

Fistula – An abnormal track between two epithelium-lined surfaces that is open at both ends.

Free tie – Single strand of suture not attached to a needle used to ligate a vessel, duct or other structure.

Granulation tissue – formation of fibrous collagen to fill the gap between the edges of a wound healing by contraction.

Hematoma – Collection of extravasated blood trapped in tissue.

Hemorrhage – A loss of gross amounts of blood in a short amount of time.

Hemostasis – The termination of bleeding by mechanical or chemical means or by the complex coagulation process of the body, consisting of vasoconstriction.

Hermetically – Sealing a package so as to make it air tight.

Herniation – A protrusion of an organ through an abnormal opening.

Hydrolosis – Decomposition or breakdown of suture with water.

Hypertrophy – An increase in the size of an organ caused by an increase in the size of the cells rather than the number of cells.

Infection– The invasion of the body by microorganisms.

Integumentary – The skin and its appendages, hair, nails, and sweat and sebaceous glands.

Intracorpeal – Something that is inside the body.

Intracuticular – Pertaining to the layers within the skin.

Intradermal – Pertaining to within the tissue of the skin.

Intrinisic – Originating from or situated within an organ or tissue.

Invert – To turn tissue inside out.

Keloidal – An overgrowth of collagenous scar tissue at the site of a wound of the skin. Dark skin is more susceptible to keloid formation.

Keratinized – Epithelial cells exposed to the external environment lose their moisture and are replaced by horny tissue.

Labyrinth – the inner package of suture material.

Ligating – The process of tying off a blood vessel or duct with a suture.

Leukocytes – A white blood cell, one of the formed elements of the circulating blood system. Leukocytes function as phagocytes of bacteria, fungi, and viruses.

Lister – Baron Joseph Lister, born in 1827, introduced the use of antiseptic surgery in a London hospital with the use of diluted carbolic acid.

Lunula – A semilunar structure, such as the crescent shaped pale area at the base of the nail of a finger or toe.

Maraging – Is two times harder than stainless steel and 85% harder than pure titanium.

Monofilament – a single strand of suture material.

Multifilament – several suture strands braided or twisted together.

Necrosis – Localized tissue death that occurs in groups of cells in response to disease or injury.

Phagocytosis – The process that certain cells engulf and destroy microorganisms and cellular debris.

Primary suture line – A line of sutures that holds the wound together during the healing process.

Radiopaque – Not permitting the passage of x-rays or other radiant energy.

Sebaceous- Fatty, oily, or greasy, usually referring to the oil secreting glands of the skin or to their secretions.

Sebum – The oily secretion of the sebaceous glands of the skin, composed of keratin, fat and cellular debris.

Seroma – Collection of extravasated serum from interstitial tissue or a resolving hematoma in tissue.

Sinus tract – A tract between two epithelium-lined surfaces that is open only at one end.

Stratum basale – The deepest of the five layers of the skin.

Stratum spinosum – One of the layers of the epidermis composed of several layers of polygonal cells.

Stratum granulosum – A layer of the epidermis, situated just below the stratum corneum except in the palms of the hands and the soles of the feet.

Stratum lucidum – A layer of the epidermis, situated just beneath the stratum corneum and present only in the thick skin of the palms of the hands and the soles of the feet.

Stratum corneum – The horny, outermost layer of the skin.

Sudoriferous – A duct leading from a sweat gland to the surface of the skin.

Tensile strength – the load per cross sectional area unit.

Tetanus – An acute, potentially fatal infection of the central nervous system caused by an exotoxin, tetanospasmin, expanded by the anaerobic bacillus, Clostridium tetani.

Tie on a passer – a free tie clamped to the tips of a forceps.

Stick tie – A single strand of suture attached to needle.

Swaged – suture permanently attached to an eyeless needle.

Tagged – the suture is secured with a hemostat or mosquito clamp and instead of being cut.

Vasoconstriction – The narrowing of the lumen of a blood vessel.

Wicking – the braided suture acts as a vehicle for organisms to move through tissue.

Index